Treatment-Resistant Schizophrenia

Stavroula Rakitzi • Polyxeni Georgila

Treatment-Resistant Schizophrenia

Evidence-based Pharmacotherapy, Cognitive Behavioral Psychotherapy and Rehabilitation

Springer

Stavroula Rakitzi
Private Practice
Athens, Greece

Polyxeni Georgila
Private Practice
Athens, Greece

ISBN 978-3-031-64622-5 ISBN 978-3-031-64623-2 (eBook)
https://doi.org/10.1007/978-3-031-64623-2

This Springer imprint is published by the registered company Springer Nature Switzerland AG
The registered company address is: Gewerbestrasse 11, 6330 Cham, Switzerland

This book is dedicated to all people with schizophrenia and treatment-resistant schizophrenia; to my patients with treatment-resistant schizophrenia; to my parents and my family; to my colleague Polyxeni Georgila; and to Prof. Dr. Annette Schröder, my supervisor in my Ph.D. studies at the University of Koblenz-Landau, Germany.

Stavroula Rakitzi

This book is dedicated to all people with schizophrenia and treatment-resistant-schizophrenia; to my patients with treatment-resistant schizophrenia; to my three daughters and to my sisters; to my parents; to my mentor Prof. E. Garelis; and to my colleague Stavroula Rakitzi.

Polyxeni Georgila

Preface

This book focuses on evidence-based interventions in treatment-resistant schizophrenia. It talks about modern and effective treatment methods performed today.

In addition, this book presents our new perspective on the therapy of treatment-resistant schizophrenia, a new treatment approach aimed at long-term recovery that combines pharmacotherapy, cognitive-behavioral therapy, and rehabilitation.

This handbook presents the results of our clinical experience with treatment-resistant schizophrenia. This group of people with schizophrenia faces many problems and frequent relapses. Therefore, it is very important to talk about a new perspective regarding the therapy of this subgroup. Our new recovery-oriented model ensures a fresh start in therapy for people with treatment-resistant schizophrenia and their families.

Mental health professionals may also find our model useful in their own clinical practice.

This book is intended for the following mental health professionals: clinical psychiatrists, clinical psychologists, and cognitive-behavioral psychotherapists, students and researchers in psychology and medicine.

Athens, Greece — Stavroula Rakitzi
Athens, Greece — Polyxeni Georgila

Introduction

Treatment-Resistant Schizophrenia: Evidence-Based Pharmacotherapy, Cognitive Behavioral Psychotherapy and Rehabilitation presents an inclusive book about one of the most difficult chronic mental health disorders, treatment-resistant schizophrenia. Evidence-based treatments, such as pharmacotherapy, cognitive behavioral psychotherapy, and rehabilitation, will be discussed. A new recovery-oriented model for treatment-resistant schizophrenia will be proposed. This book is a useful manual for experts, such as clinical psychiatrists, clinical psychologists, cognitive behavioral psychotherapists, and researchers, as well as students of psychology and medicine.

Acknowledgments

We are grateful to all of our patients suffering from schizophrenia and TRS who have participated in our treatments. We are also grateful to Dr. Sylvana Freyberg from Springer Nature and, of course, to Springer Nature.

Competing Interests We declare that we have no competing financial or non-financial interests in relation to the content of the book.

Ethical Approval We adhere to the ethical standards of the 1964 Declaration of Helsinki and its later amendments. We have included a statement that consent for publication was obtained from the participating individuals.

About This Book

Treatment-resistant schizophrenia is one of the most challenging mental health disorders and is associated with a high risk of relapse, repeated hospitalizations, suicidal behavior, and poor quality of life.

This book focuses on treatment-resistant schizophrenia, its clinical features, and evidence-based treatments: pharmacotherapy, cognitive-behavioral psychotherapy, and rehabilitation.

A novel therapy targeting long-term recovery for treatment-resistant schizophrenia is discussed. The cognitive, metacognitive, and recovery perspectives represent the main elements.

Each chapter begins with an abstract, followed by learning objectives, introduction, main text, discussion, conclusion, review questions, and bibliography. This structure, including learning objectives and review questions, reinforces the reader's learning process. It can also help improve the teaching process in seminars and courses.

Contents

About the Authors

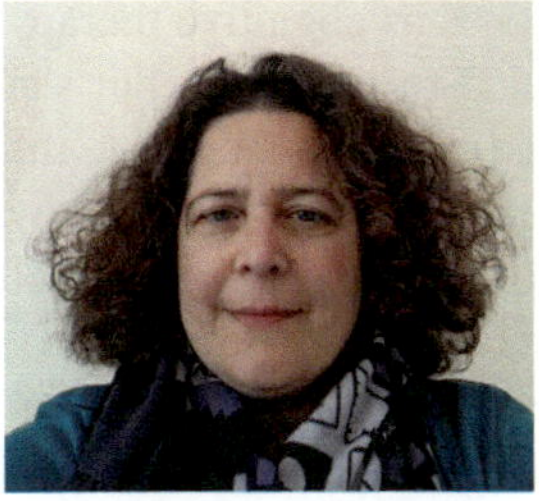

Stavroula Rakitzi completed her studies in psychology at the Georg-August University of Göttingen in Germany. She has the European Diploma in Psychology. She has completed her training in cognitive-behavioral psychotherapy in Athens according to EABCT criteria. Furthermore, she completed her Ph.D. in clinical psychology and adult psychotherapy at the University of Koblenz-Landau in Germany. Since 2001, she has worked as a Diplompsychologist and qualified cognitive-behavioral psychotherapist in private practice. She has been promoting Integrated Psychological Therapy (IPT) for individuals with schizophrenia since 2006 in Greece. She is a lecturer in cognitive behavioral therapy and in IPT at her private practice in Athens, Greece. Furthermore, she developed the IPT postgraduate program for psychologists and psychiatrists in Greece trained in CBT. She participated in many national and international conferences as a speaker and authored articles in Greek and international journals and books.

Furthermore, she is the author of the Springer Nature book *Clinical Psychology and Cognitive Behavioral Psychotherapy. Recovery in Mental Health.* She is the editor of the Greek book *Intervention in Schizophrenia. Athens: IETHS*. She is a member of the Hellenic Society for Behavioral Research and Therapy (www.eees.gr), of the Bundesverband Deutsche Psychologen und Psychologinnen (BDP) (www.bdp.org), and of the American Psychological Association (www.apa.org).

srakitzi@gmail.com.

https://www.linkedin.com/in/stavroula-rakitzi-0b512b45/

https://www.psychologenportal.de//karte/stavroylarakitzi.html

www.researchgate.net
http://orcid.org/0000-0002-5231-6619
Twitter: @SSrakitzi
Web of Science Researcher ID: AAT-7720-2020

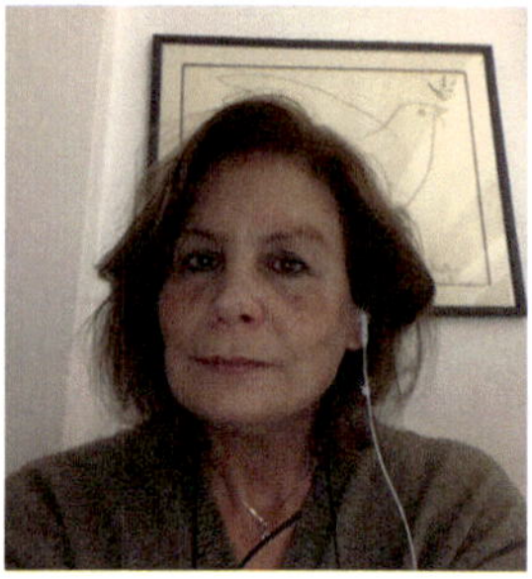

Polyxeni Georgila is a psychiatrist in private practice and the former director of the adult psychiatry department at the General Hospital "G. Gennimatas" in Athens, Greece. She completed her medicine studies at the University of Athens and specialized in neurology and psychiatry at Eginition Hospital in Athens, Greece. She completed Professor Papakostas cognitive therapy program at Eginition Hospital. Not only that, but she was trained in the psychiatric department at the Karolinska Institute in Saint Görans Hospital by Professor Wettenberg. Furthermore, she was a member of the mental health committee of the Greek Ministry of Health. Her clinical and research interests focus on all psychiatric disorders. She codeveloped the Integrated Psychological Therapy (IPT) postgraduate program for psychologists and psychiatrists in Greece trained in CBT. She has participated in many national and international conferences as a speaker and member of scientific committees, and authored articles in Greek and international journals and books.

Furthermore, she is an editor of the Greek book *Intervention in Schizophrenia. Athens: IETHS*. She is a member of the Hellenic Psychiatric Association and the Hellenic Association of Clinical Psychopharmacology.

polyxenigeorgila@gmail.com
https://gr.linkedin.com/in/polyxeni-georgila-940b521a7
http://orcid.org/0000-0003-3137-506x

Abbreviations

CBT	Cognitive behavioral therapy
CBTp	Cognitive behavioral therapy for psychosis
CT-R	Recovery-oriented cognitive therapy
MCT	Metacognitive training
MERIT	Metacognitive reflection and insight therapy
RECOVERYTRSGR	Greek recovery-oriented model for TRS
TRS	Treatment-resistant schizophrenia

List of Figures

List of Tables

1 Introduction

Schizophrenia and treatment-resistant schizophrenia (TRS) represent chronic mental health disorders associated with higher vulnerability, stigma, burden, and suicidality for individuals and their families. So it was very important for us, as mental health professionals, to publish a book that focuses on schizophrenia and TRS. These disorders deserve our attention, dedication, and willingness to conduct research protocols on the effectiveness and efficacy of evidence-based interventions as well as to implement interventions based on the evidence of these individuals and ultimately, they deserve our capability to make an appropriate diagnosis as soon as possible. All this must be done in a transparent and professional manner.

Schizophrenia and TRS present chronic mental health disorders. What does it actually means to live with a chronic mental health disorder? It means that psychiatric treatment is the basic long-term intervention. A long-term recovery-oriented psychotherapy should be an adjunctive treatment. People spend their whole lives with mental health experts, pharmacotherapy, psychotherapy, relapses, hospitalizations, and crises. It is a difficult journey. This difficult journey should be transformed into a challenge for step by-step improvement, progress, awareness, cohesion in interpersonal relationships, and a whole new meaning in life. Evidence-based recovery-oriented treatments show the way in that direction.

What TRS means? Specific psychiatric treatments are appropriate, long-term psychotherapies can address the multiple problems at the cognitive, behavioral, and emotional levels as well as at the functional outcome level. When these patients turn to us, they have already refer to many other mental health experts, have many relapses and discontinuation of their treatment, have made many suicidal attempts, or have often found themselves with suicidal ideation and they describe a general hopelessness about everything. Their cognitive deficits are a big problem for their everyday life because they cannot work, have fun and communicate with their social environment and they cannot live alone. In other words, their degree of their disability is over 80%.

S. Rakitzi, P. Georgila, *Treatment-Resistant Schizophrenia*,
https://doi.org/10.1007/978-3-031-64623-2_1

Mental health professionals are therefore required to show empathy toward patients with TRS and their families and have many years of clinical experience before trying to apply psychotherapies to them. So the most important thing for mental health experts is if we first understand in depth what TRS means.

Clinical psychiatrists, clinical psychologists, and cognitive-behavioral psychotherapists should receive appropriate training as prescribed by psychiatric societies, psychological associations, and other associations of cognitive-behavior therapy worldwide. Long-term training is always appropriate to provide information and training on evidence-based interventions.

Psychiatric conferences around the world consistently include TRS symposiums, presenting up-to-date information on the effectiveness of evidence-based interventions for TRS, and treatment complications. High suicide rates are the major problem in this disorder, and therefore it is important to make an accurate diagnosis as early as possible.

Our experience with these patients includes many cases of people going undiagnosed or being diagnosed after multiple hospitalizations. Additionally, TRS patients are often victims of negligence by mental health professionals who choose to use multiple medications with dangerous side effects or non-evidence-based psychotherapies.

TRS sufferers deserve to be able to stand up to the professional malpractices of mental health professionals in a democratic context and be treated as human beings capable of becoming active members of our society and finding their meaning to life.

This book focuses on the clinical elements of TRS, such as the diagnostic process, epidemiology, and comorbidities. Current evidence-based interventions for TRS in pharmacotherapy, cognitive-behavioral psychotherapy, and rehabilitation are discussed. A new recovery-oriented model focusing on the integration of evidence-based pharmacotherapy and psychotherapy will be presented and discussed.

The book is the result of long clinical experience and fruitful collaboration of the two authors in Greece over the years. Clinical psychiatrists and clinical psychologists providing cognitive-behavioral psychotherapy and rehabilitation to patients with schizophrenia and TRS should work together in the context of coexistence and interact for the benefit of TRS sufferers.

Long-term evidence-based pharmacotherapy and psychotherapy lead to the transformation of people suffering from schizophrenia and TRS from passive, anxious, suspicious, and weak people into dynamic individuals, more responsible and optimistic in a long-term, step-by-step dynamic change process, which leads to a better reintegration into society. Therefore, these people become active members of our society who try to be as assertive as possible about their life goals and human rights in society.

The protagonists of this book are individuals suffering from schizophrenia and TRS, as well as their families. Therefore, this book is written in such a way that not only experts but also non-specialists, like the protagonists mentioned above, can read it easily. Additionally, our work aims to protect these people from professional misconduct and abusive interventions in pharmacotherapy and psychotherapy. They may have a clear idea about evidence-based mental health interventions. Diagnosing a chronic mental health disorder presents a difficult context. It's a kind of trauma. When additional non-evidence-based interventions are implemented, a second trauma emerges, causing secondary trauma and long-term negative consequences such as stigma, social isolation, pessimism, and non-adherence to therapy. Patients lose their faith to clinical psychiatrists and clinical psychologists.

More research studies regarding the efficacy of evidence-based pharmacotherapy and psychotherapies for treatment-resistant schizophrenia are in demand. Meta-analysis, randomized controlled trials, and other types of studies regarding the efficacy of interventions by patients with schizophrenia should always clarify if the treatments are efficacious for treatment-resistant schizophrenia.

Over 30% of patients with schizophrenia belong to TRS. Therefore, published studies that include TRS are more valid and reliable regarding the reality of schizophrenia.

It is a human right to suffer from a mental health disorder such as a chronic mental health disorder, e.g., *schizophrenia and TRS; it is a human right to be vulnerable and to have access to evidence-based treatments for the best possible reintegration into society.*

Mental health experts who do not respect basic human rights of patients with chronic mental health disorders should be avoided and be under the evaluation of the ethical committees of the psychiatric and psychological associations. Patients should not be afraid and must seek for legal help from the national and international justice systems. The European Union and other countries must protect vulnerable people with mental health disorders through an international hotline and a group of scientists who will evaluate whether mental health experts have applied dangerous treatments to schizophrenia, TRS, and other mental health disorders, and shown professional misconduct.

This will be a true democratic context in which experts and scientists are evaluated throughout their whole professional careers. Experts have the power to help and to contribute to a reintegration into society but they also have the power to destroy the lives of patients with schizophrenia and TRS, if they don't follow the ethical standards of the treatments. Democracy respects and protects the rights of individuals with organic and mental health disorders.

Today we cannot assume that evidence-based interventions regarding pharmacotherapy and psychotherapy for patients with schizophrenia are not available to the scientific community and to individuals with TRS and their families.

Scientific associations offer training regarding these interventions in the context of long-term education. Participation in these trainings must be an obligation to stay updated and to offer sufferers the best possible reintegration into society. Mental health experts are responsible for the lives and dignity of the life of patients with TRS. Therefore, a long-term education of experts protects the sufferers.

Today, evidence-based interventions in pharmacotherapy and psychotherapy for TRS demonstrate that there are pathways and appropriate contexts to address the problems. This is the best response to professional misconduct, and this is why the authors want to send a key message through this book: trust evidence-based interventions regardless the difficulty of this mental health disorder.

The accessibility to empirical data regarding TRS helps us to act immediately and effectively. Time is very important to TRS treatment. By taking the appropriate therapeutical decision, we succeed in the remission of patient's symptoms and mostly decrease the suicidal risk if it exists. Empathy toward patients suffering from TRS includes a speedy cost-benefit analysis regarding a recovery-oriented treatment and appropriate psychoeducation for the patients with TRS and their families in a transparent, democratic, and professional context.

A new recovery-oriented program focusing on TRS rehabilitation will be presented and addressed. The integration of evidence-based interventions is at the forefront of this model. *This model is the result of a long-term clinical experience and the cooperation of the two authors. It includes three perspectives: the cognitive perspective-thoughts and beliefs about problems and disability; the metacognitive perspective-thoughts about thoughts and beliefs and the recovery perspective-mental health experts, and patients with TRS and their families evaluate during the whole life the impact of the evidence-based interventions throughout their lives. That means, different point of views regarding the result of psychotherapy are exchanged, and every part tries to show empathy toward the other opinion. This cohesive context helps mental health experts and sufferers to be in a dynamic and long-term process of cooperation that gives people meaning in their lives.*

Disability and problems with functional outcomes will be treated step-by-step, dynamic, problem-solving-oriented, long-term and in a democratic context, in which every opinion is important.

Our recovery-oriented model presents a new dimension in modern mental health treatment. TRS is associated with many hospitalizations, many cognitive dysfunctions, many relapses, and a high suicidal rate. Patients with TRS change very often their psychiatrists and psychotherapists. Our recovery-oriented model offers a context that gives the possibility for a long-term treatment and a safe therapeutic relationship.

Our long-term clinical experience with TRS led to the discovery of a new recovery-oriented model. Frustrations, many relapses, high suicidal risk, and many treatments without any cooperation between them are some of the problems of patients with TRS. Therefore, our recovery-oriented model tries to offer a long-term cohesive context for addressing all the problems of TRS in a stable therapeutic context.

Patients with TRS can feel safe and perceive new dimensions and possibilities in their lives when they have the chance to understand their problem with transparency and honesty, and mental health experts explain to them how the problems are expressed, how they can be coped and how important it is to be the protagonist of your own problems. Our recovery-oriented therapy follows the above mentality and structure.

Our recovery-oriented model was born in Athens Greece. Greece has been confronted with a socio-economic crisis from 2008 until today. So, this crisis and the various problems of our patients with TRS and their families have inspired us to develop such a program in a country such as Greece, which doesn't have enough invest funds in research in mental health disorders and doesn't invest also enough funds for the public mental health services. In other words, our recovery-oriented model was born and developed to address difficulties in a country that is in an on-going crisis.

It is very important to offer to vulnerable patients new opportunities regarding psychotherapy and rehabilitation. A socio-economic crisis should always be a chance to create a protective context for patients with chronic mental health disorders and their families. This means that resilience presents the best solution after a social crisis.

Our mission in the scientific community is to offer the best possible interventions for patients with TRS and their families. It is an honor for us to be part of the scientific community and to share our experience and knowledge internationally. Sharing and giving the best possible solutions to long-lasting mental health problems, such as TRS, is one of the most challenging moments for us.

The contribution of mental health specialists to the scientific community is the combination of clinical and research work, which sends multiple messages to society. This combination enables us to see how clinical practice can be evaluated through research protocols for the effectiveness of psychotherapy and pharmacotherapy.

The research protocols show us which interventions are effective, where there are problems with each treatment, and what needs to be improved in the future.

We are accountable to patients with chronic mental disorders and must provide evidence-based interventions. We are obliged to protect them from interventions that are not effective and to explain to them what is effective for their problem and what is not. Thus, patients with schizophrenia and TRS must be treated at least once a month by a clinical psychiatrist and participate in cognitive-behavioral psychotherapy and rehabilitation programs during their lives.

The implementation of non-evidence-based psychiatric and psychotherapeutic treatments is not foreseen by any scientific association nowadays. The research data on the effectiveness and efficacy of treatments for schizophrenia and TRS are indisputable. Thus, the implementation of non-evidence-based interventions is an arbitrary act and an abuse of power on the part of mental health professionals.

Evidence-based interventions meet the following criteria: they have a specific goal or goals; they have a manual that gives instructions on how the treatment can be implemented; and there are studies and meta-analyses regarding their effectiveness and efficacy. In this way, all scientists can communicate at an international level about what is effective for patients with mental disorders, especially for those with TRS and their families.

The therapeutic relationship with patients with schizophrenia and TRS has limits and goals. Any violation of these boundaries, such as establishing a personal relationship with patients, is also an abuse of power. The therapeutic relationship with patients with schizophrenia and TRS is a long-term relationship in which patients must trust and lean on therapists to initiate small and large changes in their lives.

Thus, mental health professionals are called upon to respond to this relationship by showing the limits and goals of this relationship. Any other behavior that leads to a personal and manipulative relationship with patients is an abuse of power.

Our recovery-oriented model shows how a therapeutic relationship with boundaries and goals can be built, through which evidence-based interventions can be best implemented. Finally, our model protects patients with schizophrenia and TRS and their families from abusive behaviors and abusive of power.

RECOVERYTRSGR contributes to the improvement of functional outcomes and the acceptance of the disorder. The awareness of TRS has increased. This reduces stigma, which is the worst enemy of people with chronic mental disorders and TRS. Stigma presents an aggressive behavior that leads to social isolation and the avoidance of treatments.

Finally, our recovery-oriented model shows a structured way to deal with basic problems in TRS. Each mental health expert has his/her role at different stages and is always in a cooperative relationship with the other experts. Our therapeutic gives optimistic messages and has a long-term application. It gives hope and a possibility to restart life after repeated failed treatment attempts with TRS.

The target groups for the book are students of medicine and psychology, scientists and researchers in psychology and psychiatry, clinical psychologists and clinical psychiatrists, cognitive-behavioral psychotherapists and psychotherapists, and ultimately people with TRS and their families.

Competing Interests The authors have no conflicts of interest to declare that are relevant to the content of this chapter.

Recovery in Chronic Mental Health Disorders, Especially Schizophrenia, and in Treatment-Resistant Schizophrenia

2

Learning Objectives

1. The importance of the therapeutic relationship for the recovery process in chronic mental health disorders.
2. How can we build a good relationship with people with TRS?
3. Definition of recovery.
4. The recovery process in schizophrenia and TRS.

2.1 The Recovery Process and Its Significance

Chronic mental health disorders are associated with high financial and emotional burden across the lifespan and very poor quality of life. The diagnosis of a chronic mental health disorder, such as schizophrenia, is made early in life, when individuals are young and planning their own future. Such a diagnosis constitutes an obstacle to healthy development and a sustainable future. Usually, TRS is diagnosed with a latency which differs among the cases.

The sooner evidence-based pharmacotherapy and psychotherapy begin, the better for the treatment outcome. Recovery-oriented treatment contributes to a more active role in addressing issues related to chronic mental health disorders and illness delay and prevents the onset of complex comorbidity. Recovery creates a more secure and stable future in the context of chronic mental health disorders.

Professionals, such as clinical psychiatrists, clinical psychologists, and cognitive-behavioral psychotherapists, strive to build stable, safe, long-term therapeutic relationships with patients with chronic mental disorders, such as TRS, who are in the recovery process. A long-term therapeutic relationship means a long-term commitment of the professionals to the treatment, long-term supervision as well as peer supervision of the professionals in the treatment of chronic mental disorders, and finally, proper psycho-hygiene of the experts so they can relax and take care of

S. Rakitzi, P. Georgila, *Treatment-Resistant Schizophrenia*,
https://doi.org/10.1007/978-3-031-64623-2_2

themselves. This procedure activates resources and motivates the expert to continue long-term treatment. Professionals should motivate people with TRS in every session to achieve a better quality of life and fight for their reintegration into society.

Empathy, acceptance, and positive communication are key characteristics needed to build a good long-term therapeutic relationship in the context of psychiatric treatment, cognitive-behavioral therapy, and rehabilitation. The therapeutic alliance is an important part of the therapeutic relationship and contributes to therapeutic boundaries (respect, trust, and appreciation). Four key elements are important to improve the therapeutic relationship and alliance: guided discovery through socratic questioning, consulting skills, collaborative empiricism, and case building [1]. A good long-term therapeutic relationship with TRS must be combined with the implementation of specific pharmacological and CBT interventions so that improvements can be achieved at multiple levels. A modern, evidence-based intervention must make recovery the ultimate goal of all therapies. Recovery should be assessed before, after treatment, and at follow-up several months later. In other words, recovery must be documented.

There are two definitions of recovery: recovery as an outcome (objective recovery) presents the opinions of experts and is assessed by psychometric tests. Recovery as a process (subjective recovery) represents the perspective of people with mental health disorders and their families. This opinion emphasizes the fact that the recovery process and its evaluation are dynamic and continuous. Both perspectives are important and must be considered [2].

There are many psychometric tests assessing treatment outcomes in schizophrenia and TRS, such as the Positive and Negative Syndrome Scale (PANSS) [3], Matrics Consensus Cognitive Battery (MCCB) for cognitive functions [4], WHODAS 2 0 [5, 6] for disability and functional outcomes, and recovery scales are available for process assessment. For example, *the Recovery Assessment Scale-Domains and Stages* (RAS-DS) [7–13] presents a valid, reliable, *and useful* tool for assessing recovery. *RAS-DS presents a self-report outcome measure that is translated into 18 languages. The following areas are assessed: doing things I care about, looking forward to the future, managing my illness, connecting and belonging* [7, 11, 13]. *RAS-DS is translated in Greek by Dr. Rakitzi and Mrs Sofia Katoudi (Msc). RAS-DS is used systematically by Dr. Rakitzi to evaluate the effectiveness of psychotherapy, and it will also be used also for the evaluation of the effectiveness and efficacy of RECOVERYTRSGR, as described in Chap. 4 of this book. RAS-DS presents a very interesting scale because it measures all the components of recovery and all this things that can give meaning to life. It is not only the functional outcome that is important as an outcome of psychotherapy. Recovery is also crucial as an outcome, especially when it is evaluated as a self-report.*

TRS recovery is a dynamic process that lasts throughout life. TRS patients need long-term recovery-oriented pharmacotherapy and psychotherapy.

Evidence-based pharmacotherapy is focused on the choice of the appropriate agents or the combination of them to achieve remission and recovery without dangerous side effects.

Recovery as an outcome (objective recovery) means that clinical psychiatrists should evaluate the result of the pharmacotherapy before and after 3, 6, 12, 24, etc. months from the beginning of the treatment.

Recovery as a process (subjective recovery) means that patients and their families should evaluate also subjectively the impact of pharmacotherapy and especially the side effects.

Evidence-based psychotherapy is an important complement to pharmacotherapy. Psychoeducation is the first step in helping people better understand and become more aware of this disorder. Cognitive-behavioral psychotherapy and rehabilitation improve symptoms, cognitive functioning, and functional outcomes, promoting social reintegration at multiple levels. All of these interventions contribute to remission. People with TRS should receive training in relapse prevention so they can recognize any early signs of relapse. Ultimately, recovery is the outcome and will be evaluated. This procedure is never-ending in the context of chronic mental health disorders. People with TRS and their families work together with mental health professionals.

Recovery as an outcome demonstrates the responsibility of professionals to individuals with TRS and their families. They are responsible for providing evidence-based treatments and evaluating their effectiveness and efficacy.

Recovery as a process involves the responsibility of people with TRS and their families for therapy. They should take as long as necessary to improve their symptoms and vulnerabilities; they should consult experts if they have difficulty incorporating treatments into their daily routine; and they should stand up for more rights in society under the leadership of experts.

In other words, people with TRS are protagonists, and this active role in their own problems gives them more hope for the future and strengthens their resilience. Evidence-based treatment of TRS begins with evidence-based, recovery-oriented treatments and continues with recovery (outcomes and processes) throughout the lifespan. This procedure gives people new meaning in their own lives!

The recovery perspective (recovery as an outcome and recovery as a process) offers many advantages and therefore should be taken into consideration in every evidence-based pharmacotherapy and psychotherapy. It is a democratic context in which mental health experts, patients with schizophrenia and TRS, and their families, speak openly about the positive and negative results of treatments and how the negative results can be changed. It is also a dynamic process that goes on and gives the opportunity to be evaluated in the long term. This process gives patients a new meaning in their lives and mental health experts more opportunities to increase the possibility of success by implementing interventions. Additionally, this procedure builds a cohesive context, in which experts, patients, and their families work together and respect each other. In other words, the recovery perspective fights against narcissism, arrogance, cynicism, and the indifference of the mental health experts. The recovery perspective shows the real democracy and collaboration.

The recovery perspective focuses on change, activation of resources, self-responsibility, hope, and on including new dimensions in their own lives. It is not enough to accept a difficult and chronic mental health disorder and to learn to live with it in harmony. It is necessary to change and improve the disabilities step by step, in a structured and realistic way, and to set the goal of focusing on long-term change and enhancement.

The recovery perspective has many advantages: the sufferers are the protagonists, and in collaboration with the mental health experts, the improvement is dynamic and long term so that the patients with TRS and their families can adapt to the new circumstances; only evidence-based treatments can be included; and finally, the recovery perspective guarantees protection from abusive behaviors of mental health disorders.

Mental health experts should be trained in recovery-oriented treatments. It is not enough to accept a difficult mental health disorder, such as TRS. It is necessary to bring about changes that lead to a new restart in life according to the life circumstances. This issue will be realized through recovery-oriented interventions. Change and transformation are the main important conditions for recovering from a chronic mental health condition.

The efficacy of evidence-based interventions in TRS in various settings, such as ambulant settings, hospitals, day centers, etc., *should be evaluated from a recovery perspective. Which levels of recovery has the patient of TRS achieved, and how can this prove* via *recovery as an outcome and recovery as a process? Every mental health expert should be obliged to implement recovery-oriented interventions that lead to reintegration into society in a transparent and effective way.*

Mental health experts have the power to change the lives of patients with TRS and their families. If this power is misused, the results are catastrophic for the patients. A recovery-oriented perspective and therapy display a filter between mental health experts and patients with TRS, which protects patients from misconduct and misuse. Mental health experts should be under long-lasting evaluation from the patients with TRS and their families. Patients should be assertive about every violation of their rights and every implementation of non-evidence-based interventions.

TRS looks like a complicated journey with many pathways. Some of them are easy to get; others are difficult and require attention and flexibility. It is important for the patients to live independently, with the support of mental health professionals. These procedures make patient's lives meaningful!

If the healing journey of TRS was a painting, it would have the following form: The road of the journey would be full of stones, pits, floods, and forests with wild vegetation. The evidence-based interventions would train the traveler to remove stones, avoid potholes and floods, and find paths through forests with wild vegetation. Then beautiful scenery would appear, such as a picnic in a safe place in the forest, a walk in a nice lake, and a swim in the sea. The traveler would arrive at the destination of the journey equipped to handle the difficulties while enjoying the journey.

The painting above reminds us that chronic mental disorders, such as schizophrenia and TRS, are a long journey with difficult and beautiful moments. This alternation also gives meaning to life. Difficult times and dealing with them boost our self-confidence, increase our motivation to enjoy our lives, and encourage us to continue every day to fight the difficulties but also to enjoy the small positive moments.

Our recovery-oriented treatment, which is proposed in this book and discussed in Chap. 4, looks like the painting above. Patients with TRS and their families turn the difficulties of TRS into action for life, having been trained from a recovery perspective.

Recovery is a very important point of view that we had to include. It will lead to changes and new adaptations in life. It is not enough to accept the problem and learn to manage it. We need to train the people in the recovery perspective to implement the appropriate changes as soon as possible.

Taken together, the recovery perspective and its significance were discussed, recovery was defined, and psychometric tests that evaluate recovery were presented. Finally, the advantages of the recovery process were also discussed.

2.2 Conclusions

Long-term therapeutic relationships between mental health professionals and people with TRS in recovery are appropriate so that they can feel safe and stable to continue their recovery process. The recovery as an outcome and the recovery as a process represent two perspectives, equally important to TRS.

Revision Questions

1. Why is it important to build a good therapeutic relationship in the context of the recovery of a chronic mental health disorder?
2. Which factors contribute to a therapeutically positive change in TRS?
3. Define recovery.
4. Describe the recovery process in TRS.

Competing Interests The authors have no conflicts of interest to declare that are relevant to the content of this chapter.

References

1. Kazantzis N, Dattilio FM, Dobson KS. The therapeutic relationship in cognitive behavior therapy: a clinician's Guide. New York: Guilford Publication; 2017.
2. Leonhardt BL, Huling K, Hamm JA, Roe D, Hasson-Ohayon I, McLeod HM, et al. Recovery and serious mental illness: a review of current and clinical and research paradigms and future directions. Exp Rev Neurotherapeut. 2017;17:1117–30. https://doi.org/10.1080/14737175.2017.1378099.
3. Kay SR, Fiszbein A, Opler LA. The positive and negative syndrome scale (PANSS) for schizophrenia. Schizopr Bull. 1987;13(2):261–76.
4. Nuechterlein KH, Green MF. MATRICS consensus cognitive battery. Los Angeles: MATRICS Assessment Inc.; 2006.
5. World Health Organization. International classification of functioning, disability and health (ICF). Geneva: World Health Organization; 2001.

6. Koumpouros Y, Papageorgiou E, Sakellari E, et al. Adaptation and psychometric properties' evaluation of the Greek version of WHODAS 2.0. Pilot application in Greek elderly population. Health Serv Outcomes Res Methodol. 2018;18(1):63–74. https://doi.org/10.1007/s10742-017-0176-x.
7. Hancock N, Scanlan JN, Bundy AC, Honey A. Recovery Assessment Scale-Domains & Stages (RAS-DS) manual-version 3. Sydney: University of Sydney; 2019.
8. Hancock N, the University of Sydney, Rakitzi S, Katoudi S. Recovery Assessment Scale-Domains & Stages (RAS-DS). The Greek version; 2023.
9. Hancock N, Scanlan J, Honey A, Bundy A, O'Shea K. Recovery Assessment Scale-Domains & Stages (RAS-DS): its feasibility and outcome measurement capacity. Austr New Zeal J Psychia. 2015;49(7):624633. https://doi.org/10.1177/0004867414564084.
10. Scanlan JN, Hancock N, Honey A. The Recovery Assessment Scale-Domains and Stages (RAS-DS): sensitivity to change over time and convergent validity with level of unmet need. Psychiatry Res. 2018;216:560–4. https://doi.org/10.1016/j.psychres.2018.01.042.
11. Hancock N, Scanlan JN, Kightley M, Harris A. Recovery Assessment Scale-Domains and Stages (RAS-DS): measurement capacity, relevance, acceptability and feasibility of use with young people. Early Interv Psychiatry. 2019;14:179–87. https://doi.org/10.1111/eip.12842.
12. Ramesh S, Scanlan JN, Honey A, Hancock N. Feasibility of Recovery Assessment Scale-Domains and stages (RAS-DS) for every day mental health practice. Front Psych. 2024;15:1256092. https://doi.org/10.3389/fpsyt.2024.1256092.
13. Honey A, Hancock N, Scanlan JN. Staff perceptions of factors affecting the use of RAS-DS to support collaborative mental health practice. BMC Psychiatry. 2023;23:500. https://doi.org/10.1186/s12888-023-04996-2.

Treatment-Resistant Schizophrenia

3

Learning Objectives

1. Definition of schizophrenia.
2. Definition of TRS.
3. Is TRS a distinct category?
4. Why is TRS difficult?
5. Evidence-based pharmacotherapy for TRS.
6. Evidence-based psychotherapy for TRS.

3.1 Introduction

Schizophrenia and especially treatment-resistant schizophrenia are chronic mental health disorders, which have long-term negative consequences on the quality of life and on the daily routine of the people with schizophrenia and their families. The sooner a valid diagnosis is given, the better for the person and their family.

Treatment resistance in mental health disorders is determined by the following factors: the correct diagnosis was made, appropriate treatment was proposed, but the treatment response remained inadequate. Treatment resistance is classified as primary (early onset) at the early beginning of pharmacotherapy and secondary (late onset) when an initial good response leads to an inadequate response to treatment over time [1].

A third of people with schizophrenia belong to TRS [2]. Treatment-resistant schizophrenia is defined as the persistence of positive, negative, and cognitive symptoms, although there were ≥2 trials of antipsychotic medication with the appropriate dose, duration, and adherence. TRS occurs during the first psychotic episode or may occur later in the development of the disorder [3].

The Treatment Response and Resistance in Psychosis (TRRIP) group recommended a trial of 2 antipsychotics for ≥6 weeks each at a dose equivalent to ≥600 mg

S. Rakitzi, P. Georgila, *Treatment-Resistant Schizophrenia*,
https://doi.org/10.1007/978-3-031-64623-2_3

of chlorpromazine daily as a treatment for TRS. Adherence and response to treatment should be measured in an evidence-based way.

Primary TRS is expressed at the beginning of antipsychotic medication. Secondary TRS is manifested in individuals who initially respond to antipsychotics but later become resistant [4].

The American Psychiatric Association recommends, for people with schizophrenia, evidence-based pharmacotherapy and psychotherapy. Clozapine is recommended for treatment-resistant schizophrenia (TRS), resistant suicidal behavior, and aggressive behavior in individuals with schizophrenia. Psychoeducation, cognitive behavioral psychotherapy for psychosis (CBTp), cognitive remediation, supported employment, social skills training, family interventions, and assertive community treatment are proposed as evidence-based psychotherapies [5].

The European Psychiatric Association recommends evidence-based pharmacotherapy, psychoeducation, cognitive remediation, physical exercise, social skills training, rehabilitation, and web- as well as mobile-based interventions for people with schizophrenia [6–8].

Individuals with TRS show more deficits in executive functioning, general cognitive function, attention, working memory, information processing speed, visual memory and learning, and especially in verbal memory and learning and in language functions, in comparison to treatment-responsive schizophrenia [2]. People with TRS have high rates of suicide, many comorbidities related to physical and mental health, frequent hospitalizations, more cognitive dysfunctions, and ultimately high rates of social isolation [9].

TRS can be a different illness category in comparison to treatment-responsive schizophrenia. TRS shows glutamatergic abnormalities, a lack of dopaminergic abnormalities, and important decreases in gray matter in comparison to treatment-responsive schizophrenia. Research should go on regarding the above issue [10].

Independently of whether TRS is a distinct category or not, this disorder deserves our attention and expertise in order to give the best possible evidence-based pharmacotherapy and psychotherapy.

Taken together, the main principle is that individuals with TRS don't respond positively to antipsychotic medication, and therefore the switch to clozapine or a combination of clozapine and other antipsychotic medications presents the solution to the problem of TRS. Over 30% of individuals with schizophrenia belong to TRS. That means that pharmacotherapy doesn't have a positive impact on the symptoms at the beginning. Nowadays, there are specific, well-known medications that are recommended for treatment-resistant schizophrenia. The sooner the diagnosis of TRS is given with the appropriate pharmacotherapy, the better for the person with it and their family. Treatment-resistant schizophrenia is associated with high suicidality, frequent hospitalizations, more comorbid disorders, and more cognitive dysfunctions.

All these factors lead to social isolation, very poor adherence to pharmacotherapy and psychotherapy, and decreased motivation for finding a new meaning in this life.

Polypharmacy presents a phenomenon where people with treatment-resistant schizophrenia are confronted. This situation leads to more dangerous side effects, which can cause the death of the person or lead to very bad adherence to medication and a dropout from the pharmacotherapy.

Electroconvulsive Therapy (ECT) is effective in the cases of severe depression, long-term mania, and catatonia and can also be implemented in TRS [11, 12]. *ECT can be chosen in TRS to treat clozapine-resistant schizophrenia, especially in cases of catatonia, in enormous suicide risk, or in TRS cases that need a rapid improvement because of the severity of their condition. In cases where ECT has a positive impact, it should be suggested on a maintenance basis, combined with clozapine or with other antipsychotic agents* [13, 14].

Nowadays ECT should be the last solution in very dramatic cases of TRS, as it has already been pointed it out. Our priority in TRS should always be the appropriate pharmacotherapy in safe doses combined with long-term psychotherapy.

Cognitive behavioral psychotherapists, who lack training and sufficient clinical experience in schizophrenia, are more likely to miss TRS and its negative consequences. Special training in psychotherapy is needed for people with schizophrenia and TRS to avoid unethical and evidence-free treatments.

The combination of ethical and evidence-based pharmacotherapy, cognitive behavioral psychotherapy, and rehabilitation with a recovery perspective provides a new impetus for people with TRS regarding reintegration in society and hope to improve every day.

One of the most promising things for people with TRS is the science and research involved. Life in the context of chronic mental health disorders must be approached with optimism, resilience, activation of resources, responsibility for the disorder, and faith in evidence-based pharmacotherapy and psychotherapy.

Working with chronic mental health disorders, such as TRS, is a great challenge matter. The long-term collaboration with the patients and their families led us to restructure our own beliefs as mental health experts toward schizophrenia and TRS. Patient- and structure-oriented strategies and motivation-oriented and recovery-oriented therapeutic skills are important to cope with possible frustration during the long-term therapeutic process. Additionally, mental health experts should take care of themselves and find time during the week to relax, to spend time with family and friends, and to prepare themselves for the next week with all these therapeutic sessions with sufferers of TRS. A long-term therapy for TRS means greater responsibility and cohesion, as well as step-by-step recovery on all important levels, such as cognitive, emotional, and behavioral levels, functional outcome, and quality of life.

The therapeutic relationship with TRS has two phases: The first phase is the getting-to-know-you phase, recording what has not gone well so far as well as the advantages and disadvantages of previous interventions. Thus, mental health professionals are listeners in this phase and provide a platform to express the negative thoughts and feelings of patients with TRS and their families.

Empathy toward the problems of the past is the main principle and strategy. The second part of the relationship goes into action and intervention by transparently highlighting how the treatment will be done.

Patients with TRS and their families are our close partners, without whom the treatment cannot be implemented. Intervening in the family and working with them is a very basic part of the treatment and the therapeutic relationship. In Greece in particular, the majority of TRS patients live with their families and have their financial and emotional support.

A democratic society has a responsibility to protect the human rights of all people with mental health disorders and must provide access to evidence-based pharmacotherapy and psychotherapy. People with TRS need to be doubly protected from malpractices in clinical practice, such as polypharmacy, and non-evidence-based psychotherapy.

3.2 Diagnostic Procedure

According to DSM-5-TR, at least one of the following symptoms must be present: delusions, hallucinations, disorganized speech, grossly disorganized or catatonic behavior, and negative symptoms. The person is not functional. The disturbance has been present for at least 6 months. Cognitive impairment is also a major issue and has a negative impact on the daily routine, and finally, the lack of insight into the disorder is frequently associated with poor treatment compliance [15].

A differential diagnosis should be made from major depressive or bipolar disorder with psychotic features or catatonic features, from schizoaffective disorder, from schizophreniform and brief psychotic disorder, from delusional disorder, from schizotypal personality disorder, from obsessive-compulsive disorder and body-dysmorphic disorder, from post-traumatic stress disorder, from autism, and finally from other mental health disorders with a psychotic episode [15].

Schizophrenia and TRS may coexist with a personality disorder that should be diagnosed with DSM-5-TR [15]. *Mental health experts should focus on the treatment of schizophrenia as a first priority and, secondly, of the personality disorders. It can be possible that the stabilization of TRS can lead to an improvement in the personality disorder.*

The combination of TRS and avoidant personality disorder means that the patient feels inferior to others and is very sensitive toward rejection and criticism. TRS with comorbid dependent personality disorder means that the person cannot live without having dependent relationships in which he/she feels secure and safe and disagreements are not expressed. Obsessive-compulsive personality disorder and TRS are characterized by a focus on order, perfectionism, and control.

A narcissistic personality disorder and TRS show grandiosity, want to be admired, and have lack of empathy. A histrionic personality disorder and TRS seek attention always. A borderline personality disorder and TRS show impulsivity, unstable relationships, and suicidal behavior, and feelings of emptiness. TRS and antisocial personality disorder violate the rights of others and show criminal behavior. A schizotypal personality disorder and TRS show social and interpersonal deficits, suspiciousness, and magical thinking.

A schizoid personality disorder and TRS are isolated from other people, choose solo activities, and take pleasure in few activities, and have no close friends. A paranoid personality disorder and TRS show a lack of trust toward others and suspiciousness.

A dual diagnosis of TRS and a severe personality disorder present a very difficult issue. It is well known that a severe personality disorder makes everything difficult, including the therapeutic relationship. These people have many problems building stable relationships with others, showing empathy toward others and showing respect for the rights of other people. That means that resistant positive and negative symptoms, cognitive dysfunctions, and problems with functional outcome will be treated more difficultly in combination with a severe personality disorder.

Focusing treating personality disorders as a priority would be detrimental to AS. It should therefore be emphasized that our priority is the treatment of TRS and then the issues related to personality disorders.

Psychometric scales for schizophrenia, recommended for the diagnostic procedure, are the Positive and Negative Symptoms Scale (PANSS), the scale for the assessment of positive symptoms (SAPS), the scale for the assessment of negative symptoms (SANS), the clinical global impression of schizophrenia (CGI-SCH), and the Matrics Consensus Cognitive Battery for the cognitive functions in schizophrenia [16, 17].

All the appropriate medical evaluations should be made during the differential diagnostic procedures such as blood tests, cardiological control, and electroencephalogram of axial brain or magnetic brain.

3.3 Epidemiology

The lifetime prevalence of schizophrenia is 0, 3%–0, 7%. [15]. The prevalence of treatment-resistant schizophrenia is lower than 30% in the USA or 17% in other studies [18, 19]. A younger age of onset is the most consistent risk factor for TRS [19].

3.4 Comorbidity

Comorbidity with depression, anxiety disorders, obsessive-compulsive disorders, substance use disorders, and especially tobacco use disorders as well as other medical conditions such as the metabolic syndrome or diabetes, in schizophrenia and treatment-resistant schizophrenia is very common. Finally, the risk of suicide is very high [15]. *Comorbid disorders caused by TRS should be evaluated quickly so that an appropriate therapeutic plan can include them. TRS has a very high suicidal risk, which should be treated as a first priority. The comorbid obsessive-compulsive disorders caused by TRS make everything more difficult and should be treated properly. Depression and other anxiety disorders display a common problem in TRS, and finally, patients with TRS don't take care of themselves and are frequently confronted with the metabolic syndrome.*

Comorbidity in TRS can also lead to a high morbidity risk. These people do not take care of themselves, resulting in serious organic health problems, and often have many other accompanying mental health disorders. The treatment of comorbid disorders in TRS is crucial and equally important as the treatment of TRS!

Co-occurring personality disorders should be assessed. A therapeutic plan regarding intervention for personality disorders should be realized after the main treatment for TRS. In other words, TRS is the priority of the therapy.

3.5 Evidence-Based Pharmacotherapy, Cognitive Behavioral Psychotherapy, and Rehabilitation in Treatment-Resistant Schizophrenia

Pharmacotherapy is the main therapy for patients with schizophrenia. The latest updates on pharmacotherapy for treatment-resistant schizophrenia will be presented.

Antipsychotics are effective for schizophrenia and TRS [20–23]. Pharmacotherapy showed unsatisfactory improvements regarding cognition and negative symptoms [24, 25].

Clozapine is the first treatment option for TRS [26, 27]. It is superior to other antipsychotics in improving positive and negative symptoms, overall symptoms, and relapse rates in TRS and non-refractory schizophrenia, despite the fact that clozapine is associated with some serious disadvantages [26–29]. Future clozapine studies are recommended [30].

Neurobiological findings show the difference between TRS and NTRS. Further studies should be conducted in the future [31].

Polypharmacy, which had been used to some extent in the previous years in TRS patients, turned out to be a very dangerous policy with dramatic side effects that occurred because of the cooperative activity of several agents. Side effects such as acute dystonia, tardive dystonia, tardive dyskinesia, extra pyramidal symptoms, Parkinson's disease, Parkinsonism, and neuroleptic malignant syndrome, which can cause death, should be out of our patient's lives nowadays.

The combination of more than two agents is against evidence-based pharmacological policy.

My clinical experience shows that clozapine is the first-choice agent for TRS patients. According to guidelines, a blood test, a heart and liver examination, and an EEG are required with blood monitoring every week at least for the following 3 months.

For patients who fail because of side effects (Table 3.1) to continue on with clozapine because of the appearance of myocarditis, tachycardia torsades, granulocytopenia, we may use another agent, typical or atypical, depending on the previous pharmacological history and mainly the patient's side effect profile.

So I usually turn my patients out on olanzapine 15–25 mg, or if it doesn't work, I use two agents, such as olanzapine 15–25 mg combined with aripiprazole 20–30 mg or olanzapine 15–25 mg combined with cariprazine 3–6 mg.

Table 3.1 Clozapine side effects

Hematological	Leukopenia Granulocytopenia
Cardiological	Orthostatic hypotension Widening QT Tachycardia torsades Myocarditis
Neurological	Epileptic seizures
Metabolic	Weight gain Increase of cholesterol Increase of triglyceride
Diabetes mellitus	Increase of glucose, insulin resistance

Clozapine is the prototypical atypical antipsychotic that has been used since 1960 for the treatment of schizophrenia, but as we know, it was withdrawn after reports of several deaths from neutropenia and reintroduced in the late 1980s with a restricted protocol, and nowadays, it is used in more countries for patients unresponsive to two other antipsychotics given in an adequate dose for an adequate duration after frequent blood monitoring and cardiological follow-up.

Pharmacological aspects of clozapine include low activity for the D_2 receptor, a huge activity for D_2 and D_4 and also the extrastriatal D_2 and D_3 receptors. Thus, there is a low incidence of extrapyramidal symptoms and also antagonistic activity at the 5-HT_{1A}, 5-HT_{2A}, and 5-HT_3 receptors and a_1 a_2 adrenoreceptors and H_1 which may be responsible for the sedative effects and the weight gain.

Some other side effects are hypersalivation, tachycardia, and constipation (10%) and rarely (1%) seizures and blood-reversible dysphasias (neutropenia, etc.) (1–2%).

Neutropenia and tachycardia torsades are the most serious and life-threatening side effects, both of which are reversible if they are timely diagnosed. As time progresses, the risk decreases to 0.07%. Additionally, clozapine doesn't increase serum prolactin.

After all, clozapine has been proven to be the most effective treatment for patients with schizophrenia, and furthermore, it is the only treatment for the TRS patients, leading them to an improvement of 40–70%.

To my experience, more than 35 years, clozapine is unique in relapse prevention. I can report good maintenance efficacy for those of my patients who have been proven TRS patients.

Positive symptoms, suicidality, hostility, comorbidity with personality disorders, and neurological side effects are mostly improved. Negative symptoms also show improvement after 6–12 months of treatment.

Clinical experience with clozapine over the past 30 years showed the following:

1. The faster clozapine is administered to TRS patients, the most effective could be.
2. Any trial with any antipsychotic agent except clozapine costs in remission time and maybe in the remission itself.
3. We shouldn't try as more antipsychotic agents as we can or augmentate the antipsychotic dose because it seems that the more an antipsychotic is augmented, the less effective it is in our TRS group.

So we should start clozapine administration as soon as TRS is diagnosed!

The dosage should be the lowest possibly effective, individualized for every patient in order hypotension, convulsions, sedation, and anticholinergic side effects should be avoided, and the agranulocyte cells count more than 2000/mm^3.

Previous antipsychotic agents should be gradually reduced, and clozapine should be started at 12.5 mg twice a day 2 days later, with a gradual increase in dose the following days, so we can achieve 300 mg/day in the following 2–3 weeks and, if necessary, a weekly increase of 50–100 mg.

Some patients may require higher doses, which reach 900 mg, but the middle therapeutical dose is around 450 mg.

If there is a necessity to terminate clozapine because of side effects (Table 3.1), it should be gradually reduced because of the possibility of withdrawal symptoms.

Clozapine should not be administered to patients with a history of leucopenia or agranulocytopenia that has occurred in past treatment.

In cases of granulocytopenia and neutropenia, we stop clozapine immediately and administer another medicine, typical or atypical, considering the side effects history in our patient. In a few cases, considering suicidality relapse, we may try restarting clozapine by increasing the dosage in a very slow rhythm, and we may succeed in reducing the symptoms without granulocytopenia development. The very rare development of myocarditis and tachycardia torsades demands the acute withdrawal of clozapine.

Other side effects, such as hypersalivation, need to be dealt with because they affect the patient's quality of life. Alternatively, we may decrease clozapine and combine it with another agent, such as amisulpride or try biperiden.

In my 35 years of experience, clozapine is unique in the treatment of TRS as it is also helpful in cases of neurological side effects, such as tardive dystonia and dyskinesia.

There is no doubt about its positive effect on the reduction of hospitalization and readmission after discharge and the rehabilitation of the patients.

Nowadays, there is not as much conflict about clozapine as in the past decades. Psychiatrists seem to be less anxious about the risk of administering clozapine, taking mostly the benefit of it.

One cannot understand anymore the psychiatrist's resistance in administrating clozapine, which is the first-choice medication, and it also costs much less than any other atypical antipsychotic (50% less).

I personally never regretted administrating clozapine. I always follow-up my TRS patients on clozapine with blood and heart monitoring in cases of agranulocytopenia, tachycardia, myocarditis, etc. Other agents that cause agranulocytosis should not be used.

On the contrary, I regret it a lot in a few cases that it was not enough time to achieve clozapine administration and patient's suicide, a very traumatic incidence that could have been avoided.

Clozapine is strictly contraindicated in epilepsy which is not well controlled and in serum cardiologic cases such as myocarditis, myocardiopathia, and hepatic or renal deficiency.

We should also take care about some anticholinergic side effects which are not life-threatening but are very inconvenient for people's lives, such as hypersalivation. Hypotension, and constipation are also bothersome and confirm a possible lack of compliance.

So we try to taper down the dose of clozapine, use a combination with another antipsychotic agent of the first or second generation, use biperiden in cases of anticholinergic side effects, or use an antiepileptic agent in cases of convulsions.

There should be monitoring of clozapine blood levels at least once a year, though some 150 enzymes of cytochrome P450 may augmentate clozapine blood levels.

ECT is a possible intervention as monotherapy in cases of clozapine-resistant patients or in cases of intolerance to side effects. Cognitive dysfunctions must be taken seriously into consideration and evaluated before ECT is going to be implemented. Further research regarding the efficacy of ECT in TRS is needed today [11–14].

Resistant cognitive problems present a major problem in TRS, so the decision whether ECT is going to be offered must be taken by experienced psychiatrists in a setting of a hospital with a psychiatric department.

I have worked for 30 years as a psychiatrist and as a director in an adult psychiatric department. It was not possible for our hospital to implement ECT. All TRS were treated with clozapine and other antipsychotic agents. I propose to try clozapine and clozapine with amisulpride in combination with long-term evidence-based psychotherapy to cope with the resistant positive, negative symptoms and cognitive dysfunctions. Long-term evidence-based pharmacotherapy combined with cognitive-behavioral psychotherapy and rehabilitation is a long road that takes time to pay off. One thing is certain: this path is more difficult for both patients with TRS and their families, as well as mental health experts. The interests of our patients are much more important, even if it takes months and years to achieve a very good therapeutic outcome.

A good therapeutic relationship, in which all the problems of agents and their side effects are discussed, gives psychiatrists a chance to follow in the long-term implementation of pharmacotherapy. Monthly sessions or twice a month present a solution for TRS in order to enhance the motivation for taking the agents correctly. Psychoeducation, close cooperation with family, and long-term evidence-based psychotherapy and rehabilitation present the right ingredients for successful ambulant therapy for patients with TRS.

As the director of the adult psychiatric department of the general hospital "G. Gennimatas" in Athens, Greece, I have followed the above strategy, which has been effective in all my TRS cases. It was not necessary to implement ECT. So we have to be very patient with the progress of our patients with TRS, evaluate them in long term and try to combine evidence-based interventions.

An ECT that has no success or no impact can destroy the therapeutic relationship and can be characterized as a kind of abuse. I have treated many patients with TRS who underwent ECT in other clinics in Athens and had no impact on TRS. The adherence to agents afterward was very bad; I had to hospitalize them for 3 months, and the family had lost every trust in psychiatry. Clozapine was the agent that helped them go home and to reintegrate into society step by step.

So there are always new dimensions in the therapy of TRS. A psychiatrist should exhaust every condition through a combination of evidence-based pharmacotherapy, psychotherapy, and rehabilitation in the context of a safe, long-term therapeutic relationship.

The clinical psychiatrist must be patient, prescribe stable agents appropriate for TRS, and focus not only on the quick short-term effect, but also on the stable and positive long-term good outcome. Thus, compliance with medication will be better. Patients with TRS are inspired by the stability and calmness of the psychiatrist and feel safe. We are not allowed to change the agents in a short period of time, only if it is necessary. Changes as a result of this treatment will be seen over time. Pharmacotherapy is not a championship in which one must emerge victorious. Pharmacotherapy is a mutual collaboration, in which there must be honesty, understanding of any problems, and an open channel of communication for all matters. Both sides win when one listens to the other. The above is even more important, since pharmacotherapy is the main treatment in TRS. It lays the foundations for the implementation of the rest of the effective psychotherapies.

Evidence-based psychotherapy in the context of cognitive behavioral psychotherapy should be transparent, understandable, and accessible to people with TRS. The entire process begins with a psychological assessment and an introduction to the possibilities of psychotherapy. The next step is to build a case formulation, an evidence-based hypothesis that explains simply how the problems arose, how they are sustained, and how they can be solved.

Zubin and Spring's [32] *vulnerability stress model* describes the relationship between vulnerability and stress. High vulnerability in stressful situations can lead to psychotic episodes. When vulnerability is controlled or reduced, individuals become more capable of coping with stress.

The *cognitive model* assumes that biological vulnerabilities (neurotransmitters) trigger the disorganization of cognitive functions. Stress reduces cognitive abilities, leads to problems with physical perception and thought processing, and leads to symptoms of schizophrenia, such as hallucinations and delusions [33].

The combination of the above models suggests a potential case formulation.

The availability of multiple evidence-based psychotherapies for schizophrenia and treatment-resistant schizophrenia demonstrates the existence of a scientific landscape for treating this difficult disorder.

Cognitive behavioral psychotherapy for psychosis (CBTp) [33], recovery-oriented cognitive therapy (CT-R) [34, 35], metacognitive training (MCT) (www.uke.de/e-mct, www.uke.de/mct_app) [36–38], metacognitive reflection and insight therapy (MERIT) https://www.meritinstitute.org/ [39, 40], various rehabilitation programs [41–50], recovery-oriented therapy programs, such as the illness management and recovery program (IMR) [51], psychoeducation [52], and cognitive behavioral family therapy [53, 54] present the main and most effective psychotherapies for treatment-resistant schizophrenia. Psychoeducation should be combined with the above-mentioned interventions and contributes to increased awareness and insight toward schizophrenia, which are associated with better and long-term adherence to the therapy and effective relapse prevention. A new start in life is possible when people understand their potential and vulnerability in a realistic context. In this way, it makes sense for the person to engage in evidence-based psychotherapy.

CBTp contributes to better coping with positive and negative symptoms, which reduces the distress from them, and also contributes to the improvement of general psychopathology, such as depression and anxiety, and of quality of life. The restructuring of various schemata, such as vulnerability, weakness, and control schema, represents a key element in this therapy.

Social skills training and behavior activation contribute to the improvement of negative symptoms and general psychopathology. It is very important to begin with the improvement of anxiety and depression, then focus on negative symptoms via behavior activation and social skills training, and lastly, to focus on decreasing the distress from delusional disorder and hallucinations and increasing the control of positive symptoms.

Improvements in comorbidities such as anxiety and depression, as well as negative symptoms, give people hope that they can cope with TRS. They are then better prepared to learn how to cope with positive symptoms that are very stressful.

CT-R presents the latest development of the Beck Group in the USA for serious mental health disorders. CT-R focuses on activating positive beliefs and actions in the context of a chronic mental health disorder, leading to resilience and recovery.

MCT, a metacognitive intervention, is a short-term intervention. It is a combination of CBT and rehabilitation, and it can be done in a group or individual setting. People with schizophrenia and TRS better understand the cognitive distortions associated with positive symptoms, learn to modify them, and think more realistically. This is one of the best prophylactic measures against psychotic episodes.

MERIT, a metacognitive intervention, is a long-term individual recovery-oriented therapy for individuals with psychosis with eight main principles. People have a better understanding of themselves, others, and how the two relate to each other, which contributes to more structure in life.

Rehabilitation programs for people with schizophrenia and TRS improve cognition, symptoms, and functional outcomes, which are a key to better and more realistic reintegration into life. More than 80% of people with schizophrenia and TRS experience cognitive dysfunction, such as neurocognition (processing speed, attention and vigilance, working memory, verbal memory, visual memory, and executive function) and social cognitive dysfunction (emotional processing, social cognition, theory of mind, social schema, and attribution).

These dysfunctions make people's lives very difficult during all stages of the disorder and are directly related to daily functional outcomes. Neurocognition and social cognition determine the appropriateness of behavior in response to routine stimuli.

Social cognition mediates the association between neurocognition and functional outcomes [55].

Rehabilitation must take into account many factors. The research regarding the effectiveness and efficacy of rehabilitation for people with psychosis should go on [56].

The authors have promoted Integrated Psychological Therapy in Greece, an integrative rehabilitation program for individuals with schizophrenia. Additionally, a training program for IPT for psychologists and psychiatrists who are trained in CBT is offered annually by the authors [41, 43, 44]. IPT is more effective for people with non-treatment-resistant schizophrenia than TRS. In addition, IPT also has a positive impact on TRS in terms of neurocognition, social cognition, and symptoms [44].

Dr S. Rakitzi and Dr. P. Georgila have cooperated with Prof. Volker Roder in Bern, Switzerland to promote IPT in Greece. IPT was implemented for the first time in Greece at the psychiatric department of the general hospital G. Gennimatas in Athens Greece [41, 43, 44]. *Additionally, both authors have developed a training program to IPT for clinical psychologists and clinical psychiatrists in Greece, who have been trained in cognitive behavioral psychotherapy and have a minimum of 3 years clinical experience with patients with schizophrenia. This trainings program lasts 1 year with 200 h of training. It focuses on education in the 5 subprograms of IPT (cognitive differentiation, social perception, verbal communication, social skills, and problem-solving). This part is very praxis-oriented, and many roles playing are going to be offered. Afterward research studies regarding IPT and schizophrenia are presented and discussed in a journal club. Finally, a research protocol regarding the implementation of IPT in the work environment of the colleagues is being offered, discussed, and supervised. We focus especially on the problems with the implementation of IPT in TRS. Our clinical and research experience has shown that IPT can be effective in TRS as well.*

IPT has many advantages: it is an integrative, evidence-based rehabilitation program that focuses on the main problems of schizophrenia, such as symptoms, cognitive functions, social skills, and problem-solving. It can last 50 sessions, which means that patients with TRS have enough time to integrate into their daily routine what they have learned in the therapy. Finally, it is implemented in a group setting, which is a very interesting learning experience.

Group therapy, especially for patients with TRS, has many advantages as an intervention framework. Members learn from each other; the group is a representation of society and the rules that apply; members obey the rules of the group and learn to work together for a purpose. IPT emphasizes to patients with TRS that it is important to try to practice and cooperate in a specific context; we do not play championships, and we do not strive for the perfect result.

Group therapy is a comprehensive learning process, in which there is an introduction to something processing and problem-solving. We listen carefully to others, take a position on what we hear, and justify our own point of view. Thus, in a group therapy like IPT, all cognitive functions, communication and expressiveness, and the way of thinking as well as the positive and negative symptoms, are improved. Thus, patients with TRS can better integrate into society and improve their quality of life and functional outcomes.

Our Greek training program for IPT gives you the chance in 200 h to understand the main principles of IPT, to discuss potential problems by implementing it for the first time, and to conduct potential research regarding the effectiveness and efficacy of IPT in Greece. We have trained in the last years some very competent colleagues in Greece in IPT, who implement it in their own clinical work environments. The training in IPT enhances the possibilities for treatment success for patients with TRS. IPT is the last year's well known in Greece, and we continue to implement it in our own private practice.

Colleagues who have been trained by us gained access to an efficacious and internationally recognized rehabilitation program for patients with schizophrenia that was implemented in their department. This way contributed to the fact that many patients with schizophrenia in Greece had the opportunity to participate in such a program.

In other words, our training program has brought IPT to many patients with schizophrenia. It is also clear that without professional training in CBT and IPT, it is very dangerous to implement such a difficult rehabilitation program.

IMR combining psychoeducation and CBT improves treatment adherence, while also providing training in social skills, management of treatment-resistant symptoms, and relapse prevention.

Cognitive behavioral family therapy, which assesses family dynamics, reduces critical comments or excessive emotional involvement of members in people with schizophrenia, improves communication between them, and restructures the dysfunctional patterns of family members.

Taken together, psychoeducation improves understanding of schizophrenia and TRS. CBTp decreases the distress from symptoms and improves the quality of life and the ability to cope with schizophrenia. CT-R strengthens particularly positive beliefs, which contribute to enhanced resilience. Rehabilitation improves symptoms and cognitive functions, promoting social reintegration. Metacognitive therapies, such as MCT and MERIT, focus on thinking about thinking, leading to intellectual distance from oneself and others while enhancing a new, more realistic perspective on life. IMR is a combination of psychoeducation, CBT, social skills, and relapse prevention to increase recovery.

Finally, cognitive behavioral family therapy will improve the family climate by reducing the negative emotions strongly expressed toward members with schizophrenia (Figs. 3.1 and 3.2).

Efficacy and effectiveness studies demonstrate that the above therapies are the treatment of choice for individuals with schizophrenia and TRS [41–61].

The question is what needs to be improved for TRS? It takes longer to build a positive therapeutic relationship with these people. They feel insecure and mistrustful and experience positive and negative symptoms of resistance as well as cognitive dysfunction. They should take as much time as necessary to feel safe before proceeding with psychotherapy. The majority of them are mistreated through the use of various drugs or ineffective psychological therapies. In other words, they have lost faith in mental health professionals and are frustrated about everything. This stage increases the likelihood of isolating oneself with the burden of stigma and dying by suicide.

Motivational interviewing [62] contributes to better preparation before starting a psychotherapeutic intervention. The family of a person with schizophrenia must be involved at this stage and play an active role in strengthening the person's motivation.

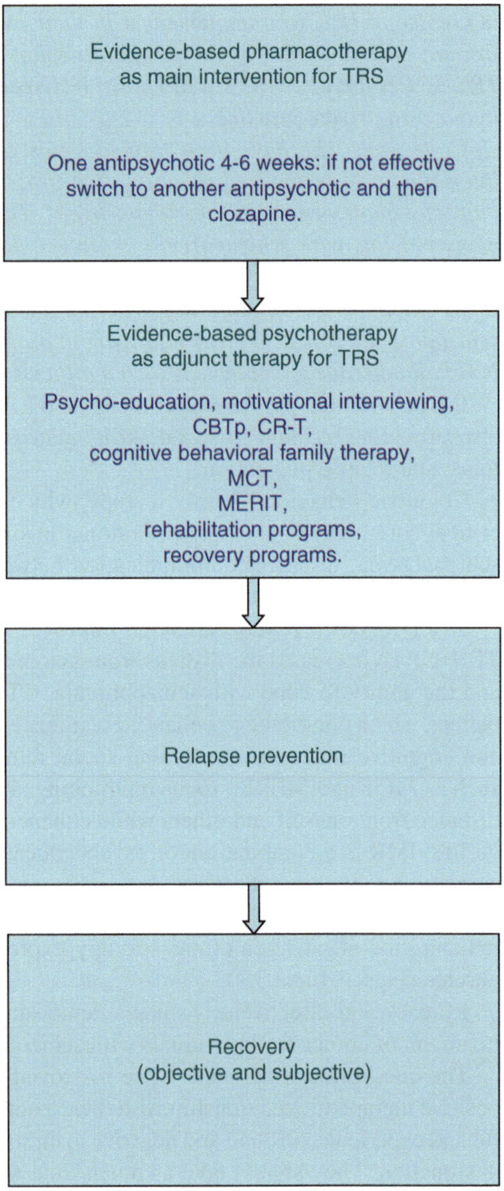

Fig. 3.1 The context of evidence-based pharmacotherapy and psychotherapy for TRS

TRS requires long-term, recovery-oriented psychotherapy. Interventions should be combined [63, 64] to ensure recovery. Finally, a close therapeutic relationship is a very important issue in the treatment of TRS [65].

Dr. Stavroula Rakitzi and Dr. Polyxeni Georgila M.D. are conducting a research protocol regarding the efficacy and effectiveness of a combination of pharmacotherapy, IPT and MCT in people with schizophrenia and TRS in Greece (clinical

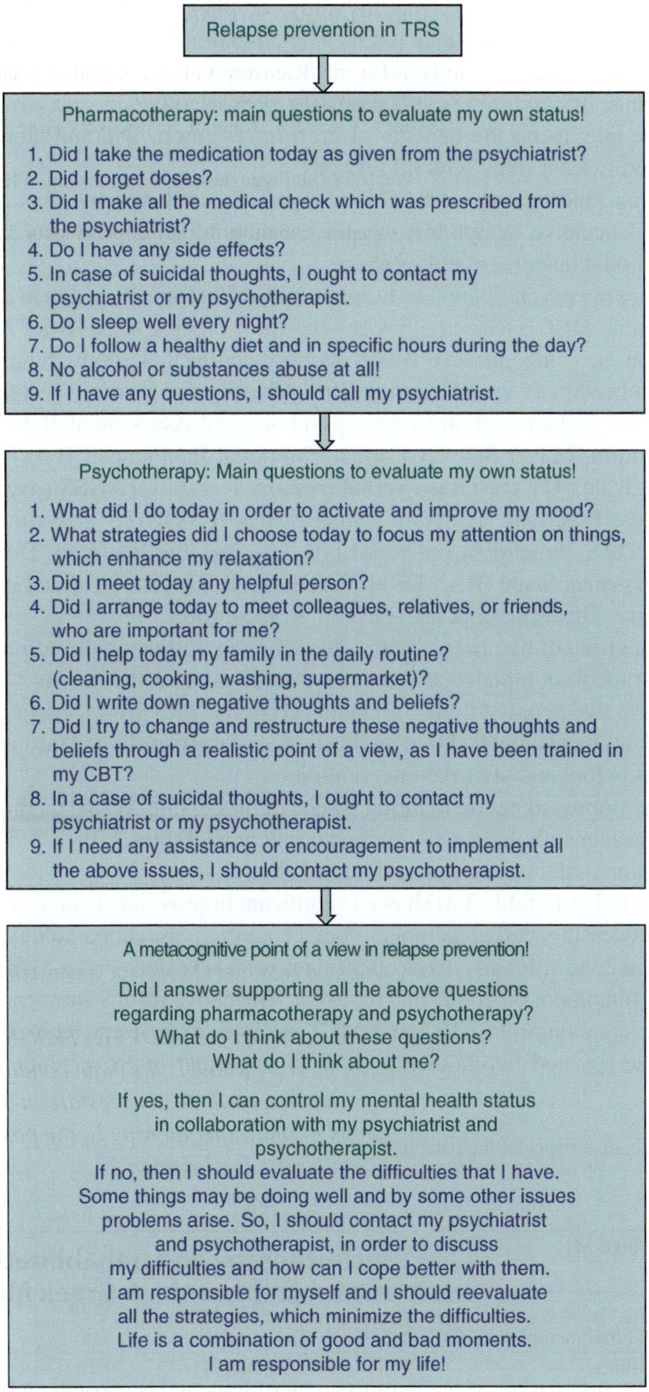

Fig. 3.2 A metacognitive model of relapse prevention in TRS. Responsibility to myself

trial registration NCT (05623228). This study complies with the ethical standards of the 1964 Declaration of Helsinki and its later amendments [66].

This protocol is being rolled out for the first time in Greece and will demonstrate the importance of combining evidence-based pharmacotherapy and psychotherapy for these people, using the benefits of each intervention. IPT and then MCT are implemented twice a week with 60 sessions.

It is a non-randomized study. This recovery-focused therapy aims to improve positive and negative symptoms, cognitive function, social and problem-solving skills, functional outcomes, and recovery.

The following psychological tests are performed before, after, and in a follow-up after 6 months: MCCB (Speed of processing (trail-making test), (Brief Assessment of cognition in schizophrenia BACS symbol-coding), working memory-verbal (Letter-Number-Span), visual learning (Brief Visuospatial Memory Test (BVMT-R), reasoning and problem-solving (Neuropsychological Assessment Battery (NAB), social cognition (Mayer Salovey Caruso Emotional Intelligence Test) [12], Social Perception Scale [41], the Greek verbal memory test [67], PANSS (psychopathology) [68], the Psychotic Symptom Rating Scales (PSYRATS) (psychopathology) [69], WHODAS (functional outcome) [70, 71], and the Recovery Domains and Stages Assessment Scale (RAS-DS) [72, 73]. WAIS [74] is performed once before the procedure. This is an ongoing research protocol [66].

The pilot group of five people with schizophrenia, following the current ongoing research protocol, completed 60 treatment sessions, and the results will be presented. These five people (Table 3.2) belonged to the TRS group, they were single, and all took atypical antipsychotic medication, and were evaluated through psychological tests before and after the intervention.

They had improved neurocognition (speed of processing, verbal memory), social cognition, psychopathology, and functional outcome (Tables 3.3).

Furthermore, effect sizes were calculated (Fig. 3.3):

The T-paired test (Table 3.3) showed significant improvements in neurocognition (speed of processing, verbal memory), social cognition, psychopathology, and functional outcome. Additionally, large effect sizes were revealed (Fig. 3.3) in cognition, symptoms, functional outcome, and recovery. The above results show the effectiveness of the combination of IPT and MCT in TRS. Long-term recovery-oriented pharmacotherapy and psychotherapy lead to important improvements, which are

Table 3.2 Characteristics of the patients

N = 5			
	M (SD)	t/chi.Sq.	*p*
Sex (40% F, 60% M)	1.60 (0.54)	5.00	0.28
Age	28.40 (5.77)	11.00	0.00
IQ	82.60 (4.77)	38.68	0.00
Employment 60% unemployed, 40% students	2.40 (0.54)	5.00	0.28
Duration of illness	12.00 (2.91)	9.20	0.001
Medication (chlorpromazine equivalents)	580.00 (349.28)	3.71 (4)	0.02

Table 3.3 T-paired test

N = 5			
	M(SD)	*t*(df)	*p*
Speed of processing			
Speed before	54.20 (4.76)		
Speed after	46.80 (9.65)	2.76 (4)	0.05
Verbal memory oral semantic			
VMO before	12.46 (0.96)		
VMO after	15.33 (1.97)	4.03 (4)	0.01
Verbal memory oral phonological			
VMO2 before	11.86 (1.65)		
VMO2 after	13.60 (1.81)	3.33 (4)	0.02
Social cognition			
SPS1 before	38.40 (13.27)		
SPS1 after	87.00 (9.35)	6.96 (4)	0.02
SPS2 before	56.00 (13.69)		
SPS2 after	79.80 (12.79)	4.88 (4)	0.00
MSCEIT before	71.60 (1.14)		
MSCEIT after	82.20 (1.30)	12.15 (4)	0.00
Psychopathology			
PSYRATS delusions			
PSYRATS D before	19.20 (4.38)		
PSYRATS D after	11.80 (3.70)	3.76 (4)	0.02
PANSSTOTAL before	107.80 (14.16)		
PANSSTOTALB after	73.80 (18.07)	6.92 (4)	0.02
Functional outcome			
WHODAS total before	49.68 (14.29)		
WHODAS total after	30.94 (7.21)	4.20 (4)	0.01
Cognitive function, communication			
WHODAS1 before	52.00 (19.87)		
WHODAS1B after	28.00 (12.54)	3.44 (4)	0.02
Social relationships			
WHODAS4 before	74.99 (20.41)		
WHODAS4B after	29.33 (13.82)	0.34 (4)	0.01

$p \leq 0.05$
Note: *SPS* social perception scale; *MSCEIT* Mayer Salovey Caruso Emotional Intelligence Test; *VMO* verbal memory oral; *PSYRATS D* psychotic symptom rating scales, delusions

associated with the reintegration of those people into society. The following impressions of this therapy were reported by all five participants: My motivation for life has increased, my communication skills, mood, and memory have improved, stress has decreased, and finally, my cognitive functions, such as concentration and memory, have improved. We want to try to work in the future.

Empirical data from the above research protocol with all the participants [65] will be published after the procedure is completed. This combination of IPT and MCT focusing on long-term recovery should help, especially TRS. Reintegration into society will be easier for participants.

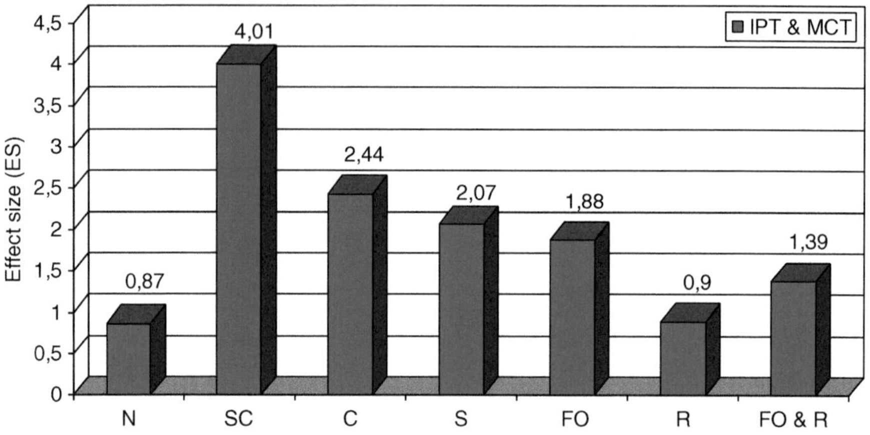

Fig. 3.3 Effect sizes in the therapy phase (T1–T2; 60 sessions): areas of cognition, symptoms, functional outcome, and recovery. Note: *N* neurocognition; *SC* social cognition; *C* cognition; *S* symptoms; *FO* functional outcome; *R* recovery; *FO & R* functional outcome and recovery

Education about relapse prevention is important in pharmacotherapy and psychotherapy. People with TRS learn to assess their own mental health and cope with changes that may contribute to relapse. It is very important to take medication as prescribed by your psychiatrist. What's the problem if you miss a dose or take more medicine? If some side effects occur suddenly, what should you do? It is very important to contact a psychiatrist immediately. If anxiety or depression occurs, take steps to reduce it, such as doing mood-boosting activities or playing sports. If hallucinations or delusions are prominent throughout the day and increase anxiety and depression, interventions should be implemented to address hallucinations or reallocate delusional thinking and any negative thoughts related to it (Fig. 3.2).

Recovery as an outcome or objective recovery means that people with TRS must be assessed using psychological testing before, after, and during a follow-up period of 6 months or more after the end of treatment. Test results must reflect changes (positive, negative, or no change) after treatment and follow-up.

Recovery as a process or subjective recovery means therapy is a dynamic and ongoing procedure rather than static. Individuals must take responsibility for their own mental health and be protagonists. It is possible that people with TRS will receive better psychoeducation after therapy about their problems; they reduce anxiety, depression, and distress and improve social skills, but they need more time to cope effectively with hallucinations and delusions.

Some days are easy, and some days are very difficult to manage. The cognitive restructuring of delusional thoughts, vulnerability schema, and control schema regarding the hallucinations requires more training and more time. Even if some problems occur, individuals can still continue their lives by working, studying, or seeing friends and family.

In summary, pharmacotherapy is the main therapy for TRS. Clozapine and other antipsychotic agents are the treatment of first choice. Pharmacotherapy should be

combined in long term with psychoeducation, cognitive behavioral psychotherapy, metacognitive training, cognitive behavioral family therapy, and recovery-oriented cognitive therapy. All the above interventions should be implemented in a context of a long-term therapeutic relationship in a stable and secure context. Psychiatrists should be very careful with ECT and should follow the guidelines of the international psychiatric associations.

3.6 Case Studies

Our case studies comply with the ethical standards of 1964 Declaration of Helsinki and are later amendments and are presented with permission from TRS sufferers. Basic information has been changed to protect individual privacy.

Sofia is 24 years old and studying history. She started psychotherapy with Dr. Stavroula Rakitzi in September 2022 and wanted to learn how to cope with anxiety. She has very good knowledge about schizophrenia and talks openly about it. Additionally, she is being treated by a private psychiatrist. She was hospitalized three times after three psychotic episodes in two different psychiatric wards. She takes many medications and experiences many side effects from polypharmacy. Dr. Rakitzi started with psychoeducation.

Her parents divorced, but they independently took very good care of their daughter. Dr. Rakitzi worked well with both parents and offered them psychoeducation about schizophrenia.

Sofia participated in individual CBTp with Dr. Stavroula Rakitzi from September 2022 to December 2022, doing 20 sessions. This individualized treatment focuses on psychoeducation in TRS, on suicidal thoughts, depression and anxiety, as well as on the control of positive symptoms (hallucinations and delusions), thus allowing these symptoms to be better controlled. Dr. S. Rakitzi referred Sofia to Dr. Georgila in September 2022 to better manage the side effects of polypharmacy. Side effects can negatively impact psychotherapy, increase medication noncompliance and suicidality, and increase stigma and social withdrawal.

For 2 years, Sofia was treated with quetiapine 200 mg, risperidone 12 mg, and biperiden 4 mg because of extrapyramidal side effects, combined with perphenazine 8.20 mg for 6 months, changed to quetiapine 600 mg, combined with stelazine 10 mg and then with quetiapine and aripiprazole without any improvement of her positive or negative symptoms.

On the contrary, she had all the side effects, such as extrapyramidal symptoms, weight gain (more than 20 kg), tremor, dyskinesia, akathisia, and prolactin elevation.

Taking into account the poor degree of symptom response, the experience of side effects, and basically the fact that Sofia was a TRS patient, clozapine was the first-choice medication.

She and her parents were informed about clozapine, its effects, and its side effects, and they agreed to administer it. After the essential blood monitoring test, the cardiological examination, and the EEG examination, Sofia was treated with clozapine with a good response of 400 mg and a full remission of auditory hallucinations, persecutory delusions, and suicidal ideation. Unfortunately, anticholinergic effects, such as hypersalivation and hypotension, occurred and to treat these side effects, clozapine was diminished to 200 mg and amisulpride was co-administered at a dose of 200 mg. The symptom remission was sustained, and the reduction of side effects was achieved.

Sofia also participated in 60 sessions of the study protocol, in which IPT was combined with MCT, from November 2022 to June 2023. This therapy focuses on positive and negative symptoms, cognitive function, social and problem-solving skills, cognitive distortions of positive symptoms, functional outcomes, and recovery.

Sofia was improved after 30 sessions of intensive psychiatric treatment and 80 sessions of recovery-oriented psychotherapy in speed of processing, problem-solving, social cognition, psychopathology, functional outcome, and recovery (Tables 3.3, 3.4, and 3.5).

She continues to receive outpatient psychiatric treatment once a month by Dr. P. Georgila and attend psychotherapy sessions of Dr. S. Rakitzi whenever she wants.

Sofia and her parents are very proud of this progress and the fact that she has found a new meaning in her life. She fought against TRS with dignity, patience, and hope. Sofia is taking a break from studying history and doesn't know if she will continue studying. Not only that, she will reassess her motivation to study in a few months. The university knew about her mental health issues. Sofia is about to have a long summer vacation and plans to work in the future. Recovery is underway!

Sofia has composed a letter to schizophrenia and treatment-resistant schizophrenia.

Table 3.4 Results of recovery-oriented pharmacotherapy and psychotherapy-cognitive functions

Evaluation	Speed of processing MCCB	Working memory MCCB	Verbal memory Greek verbal memory test	Problem-solving MCCB NAB	Visual memory MCCB	Social cognition MCCB MSCEIT	Social cognition Social perception Scale SPS A
11 2022	54	15	12.33	19	10	70	58
6 2023	44	17	13.66	11	27	83	82

Note: *SPS* social perception scale; *MSCEIT* Mayer Salovey Caruso Emotional Intelligence Test; *VM* verbal memory; *PSYRATS D* psychotic symptom rating scales, delusions

Table 3.5 Results of recovery-oriented pharmacotherapy and psychotherapy-psychopathology, functional outcome, and recovery

Evaluation	Psychopathology PSYRATH H	Psychopathology PSYRATH D	Psychopathology PANSStotal	Functional outcome WHODAS total	Recovery RAStotal
11 2022	37	24	123	67.39	101
6 2023	15	13	103	40.58	118

Note: *PSYRATS D* psychotic symptom rating scales, delusions; *PSYRAT H* psychotic symptom rating scales, hallucinations

Dear Schizophrenia,

I keep in mind me living with you from a young age. I was anxious, I couldn't sleep, I heard voices, and I was always under threat. I was very angry about this circumstance, and I didn't know what it was! Furthermore, I can portray it like numerous wild waves inside me night and day.

Psychiatrists educate me to understand what schizophrenia is. It was self-evident for me, at 18 years old, that I was mentally ill. I wanted to die by suicide. I was hospitalized three times, and it was clear for me that I am not progressing to discover a way to coexist with schizophrenia and to discover a new meaning in my life.

After the final hospitalization, I met a psychiatrist, who treated me for 5 months. He prescribed me a lot of medication and changed the medications and doses nearly every week. I had a parcel of side effects, and I needed to rest all day. This is often not life. I wanted to die by suicide.

My parents helped me find a new clinical psychologist and cognitive behavioral psychotherapists. I met Dr. Rakitzi, who begun with a psychoeducation with respect to schizophrenia. We learned together how to manage with resistant suicidality, how to cope with negative thought, with voices and how to diminish anxiety and improve depression.

Dr. Rakitzi alluded me to Dr. Georgila. I needed to visit another psychiatrist, to arrange to be treated as a human being! It was clear to me during the therapy that the side effects of medication, as explained to me by my new psychiatrist, Dr. Georgila, led to a bad quality of life. Under these circumstances, I learned a new word: treatment-resistant schizophrenia. I suffer from a treatment-resistant schizophrenia.

Medication was not so effective for my positive and negative symptoms and my cognitive functions. Clozapine was the most suitable pharmacotherapy for me! I interrupted some days of my pharmacotherapy with mini-relapses. Now, I learned that stable pharmacotherapy will improve better my symptoms and my social behavior in a long term.

The new pharmacotherapy—individual and group cognitive behavioral therapy— helped me find a new meaning in my life. I learned to acknowledge my mental health disorder, and I attempt to reschedule my life and to follow goals that will not destroy my mental health. My memory is improved, I can control my voices and delusions, my negative symptoms are also improved, and I enjoy a better life with more social interactions. I found a new meaning in my life, although I suffer from a very difficult mental health disorder with a high percentage of disability!

I would like to send a message to all the people in this world, who endure from treatment-resistant schizophrenia: We are all human beings, and we merit dignity, effective treatments, and mental health experts with transparent and human behavior. Believe in evidence-based therapies.

Marios is a 72 years old man, a widow with a daughter, and has suffered from since he was 30 years old, with intent auditory hallucinations and a persecuted delusion. He was administrated by previous psychiatrists with first-generation antipsychotic medication (haloperidol, zuclopenthixol) for two decades with side effects such as dramatic chronic dystonia and dyskinesia, which cost him a bad quality of life and insomnia because of the illness, plus anterocollis, a very painful side effect. Besides, the stigma costed him a total social isolation for most of his life.

The termination of the first-generation antipsychotic medication and the administration of clozapine about 2 months later led to the remission of auditory hallucinations, and the every 4 months botulinum toxin injection reversed gradually the anterocollis which obtained him at last after so many years of suffering to breathe and sleep properly as well as to swallow.

Thus, he and his family were very grateful for the rest of his life.

As a conclusion, clozapine has a strong effect on positive symptoms of TRS, and it seems that it affects the reversion of torticollis. PANSS [67] and WHODAS [69, 70] were administered in November 2023 (PANSS: positive symptoms 15 low, negative symptoms 18 middle, general psychopathology 37 middle, total 70 low, WHODAS total 45).

Nikos is 32-year-old man, a graduate of the third education level without a job, not married and without children. He presented with nervousness, anxiety, insomnia, and obsessive-compulsive symptoms during early adolescence. Before the first psychotic episode with auditory hallucinations, confusion, and hostility, and after the remission of the episode, he had depersonalization and derealization symptoms, referential thoughts, and social isolation, followed by the next relapse with another treatment-resistant episode, followed by the next relapse with another treatment-resistant episode, followed by negative symptoms and increased obsessive-compulsive symptoms.

The administration of clozapine achieved full remission of the positive symptoms. Additionally, he participated in our recovery-oriented psychotherapy with IPT and MCT, consisting of 60 sessions (Table 3.3, Fig. 3.3), and improved in cognitive functions, symptoms, functional outcome, and recovery. He completed his studies at the university and now is trying to find a job.

Elena is a 42-year-old woman diagnosed at the age of 25 as TRS with a history of abuse of cannabis, opioids, cocaine, and ecstasy and progressing psychotic signs such as suspiciousness, family and social isolation, which was followed by a psychotic outbreak with delusions of grandiose and the belief that she is a millionaire's daughter and has a great mission.

She had many admissions during one of them was pregnant on third month and was diagnosed also HIV positive.

She and her family wanted to keep the baby away from any risks (HIV, substance abuse, administration of methadone, and the antipsychotic medication).

She was in the hospital for 3 months. She was administered olanzapine 20 mg, and the pregnancy was successfully completed. Her mother took the responsibility for both the patient and her baby.

The follow-up is unfortunately inadequate, and she is instantly under the influence of substances.

Because of the unstable compliance and poor insight, the administration of clozapine was unfair and prohibitive. So olanzapine long-acting was the medication of choice.

Elena continues to live with her parent's family and her son, having frequent relapses and psychotic episodes and a recent suicide attempt. In other words, she is accidentally alive. PANSS [68] and WHODAS [70, 71] were evaluated (PANSS: positive symptoms 38 very high, negative symptoms 45 very high, general psychopathology 75 very high, total 158 very high, WHODAS total 85).

To conclude, in this case, therapeutic commitment is very difficult as a result of her personality as well as the consequences of the illness (cognitive and social degradation). Clozapine could be the indicated medication in the case of Elena, if she could commit herself to fixed-out follow-ups.

Psychiatrists should focus more on the behavioral disorders and less on the symptoms and the administration of first-generation antipsychotics that had so many extrapyramidal side effects and akathisia which affected compliance.

Nevertheless, there is an amount of TRS patients, maybe 30%, that are treatment-resistant to clozapine, and we must turn back to any medication that can be helpful.

So long-acting olanzapine (450 mg/month) became the alternative medication, combined with zuclopenthixol (20 mg/24 h).

Alexandros is another case, 35 years old, in which Dr. Georgila and Dr. Rakitzi have coordinated with each other in order to arrange better remission and reintegration into society. Alexandros belongs to treatment-resistant schizophrenia and schizoid personality disorder. He was hospitalized three times after psychotic episodes. Dr. Georgila has been responsible for the psychiatric treatment since 2009 until nowadays. He has been on clozapine (300 mg) the last 15 years. Dr. Georgila executed psychoeducation by the family of the patient. Alexandros participated in 20 sessions in the cognitive part of IPT therapy (cognitive differentiation, social perception, and verbal communication) between December 2010 and February 2011, which were offered by Dr. Rakitzi and Dr. Georgila. Working memory, social cognition, and negative symptoms were improved [41].

The parents of Alexandros contacted Dr. Rakitzi in December 2014, expressing their worries about his social isolation. The father had health problems, and Alexandros was very anxious about them. I proposed an individual cognitive-behavior therapy. CBTp [33] was implemented between January 2015 and October 2015 with 40 sessions, in which we focussed on psychopathology and social skills training. The improvement of negative symptoms was an important priority. Alexandros started to talk transparently about his worries regarding the health of his father. He heard voices about the big possibility of the death of his father and was not able to rest at night. He spent more time with him in social circumstances, meeting friends of his father with him. This led to the fact that he was happy about it, that he contributed to the happiness of his father, and that he learned not to center on the voices with respect to the father.

He traveled abroad with his mother, visiting friends, and he learned to be more mindful with activities at home (cleaning, shopping, etc.), appearing more empathy toward the parents, who were getting older. Finally, he reconnected with a friend from the school, meeting him every 15 days every month. After therapy, positive and negative symptoms and psychopathology, as well as social skills, made strides.

Costas is 35 years old. He has been under psychiatric treatment by Dr. Georgila the last 20 years on clozapine (150 mg). He suffers from treatment-resistant schizophrenia. Likewise, he was hospitalized twice in the past, and for the last 17 years, he has been treated ambulant by Dr. Georgila. His parents suffer from obsessive-compulsive disorder and obsessive-compulsive personality disorder, and his brother also suffers from treatment-resistant schizophrenia. Costas participated in 20 sessions in the cognitive part of IPT therapy (cognitive differentiation, social perception, and verbal communication) between December 2010 and February 2011, which were offered by Dr. Rakitzi and Dr. Georgila. Working memory, social cognition, and negative symptoms were improved [41].

Marianna is 39 years old. She was hospitalized three times after psychotic episodes. She suffers from treatment-resistant schizophrenia and has expressed a great amount of aggression under the guidance of delusions and hallucinations. Her mother died from cancer when Marianna was 17 years old. This was the beginning of psychotic episodes. She is on clozapine (100 mg) the last 15 years. Dr. Georgila implemented psychoeducation by the family of the patient and tried to progress the relationship between Marianna and her sister. Marianna was very jealous toward her sister, with many delusions.

Dr. Georgila worked intensively with her and the family to reduce this jealousy. Afterward, Marianna participated in 20 sessions in the cognitive part of IPT therapy (cognitive differentiation, social perception, and verbal communication) between December 2010 and February 2011, which were offered by Dr. Rakitzi and Dr. Georgila. Working memory, social cognition, and negative symptoms were improved [41]. She finished her studies and took on more responsibilities in the daily routine, helping her father with home activities, such as shopping and cleaning.

Additionally, she participated in our recovery-oriented psychotherapy with IPT and MCT, consisting of 60 sessions in 2023 (Table 3.3, Fig. 3.3) and improved in cognitive functions, symptoms, functional outcome, and recovery. She is now trying to discover a part-time job. Recovery is in process.

Stefanos is 26 years old and studies French philology for the last 12 years. He suffers from treatment-resistant schizophrenia. He is on clozapine (250 mg), 400 mg valproate natrium (400 mg), and cariprazine (3 mg).

Dr. Georgila treated Stefanos over 12 years monthly and implemented psychoeducation by the family of the patient. Dr. Georgila worked intensively with the family, helping Stefanos deal with the divorce of his parents, the cancer of his brother and the cancer of his mother. Stefanos was under systematic cognitive behavioral psychotherapy for 1 year in 2022 with Dr. Georgila. He improved his symptoms and social skills.

Moreover, he participated in our recovery-oriented psychotherapy with IPT and MCT, consisting of 60 sessions in 2023 (Table 3.3, Fig. 3.3), and improved in cognitive functions, symptoms, functional outcome, and recovery. He tries now to finish his studies and to distribute poems in Greek and French language. Recovery is in process.

Fani is 32 years old and suffers from treatment-resistant schizophrenia and schizoid personality disorder. She has been treated by Dr. Georgila the last 12 years and takes olanzapine (20 mg). CBTp [33] was implemented between October 2014 and October 2015 with 40 sessions, in which we focused in psychopathology and social skills training. Positive and negative symptoms were improved.

Dr. Georgila tried to endorse clozapine in 2022, which improves symptoms. Clozapine has been hindered by Dr. Georgila due to the undesirable side effects of clozapine.

Moreover, she participated in our recovery-oriented psychotherapy with IPT and MCT, consisting of 60 sessions in 2023 (Table 3.3, Fig. 3.3), and improved in social cognition, memory and in negative symptoms.

Theodora was treated by Dr. Georgila from 1990 to 2011. She suffered from treatment-resistant positive and negative symptoms and cognitive functions. She heard voices and described erotic delusions. Her father had an atypical psychotic disorder, and her mother had an obsessive-compulsive personality disorder. Theodora was also sexually abused by a psychiatrist, which was confirmed from her mother. This factor led to many psychotic episodes and a lack of trust in mental health experts.

Theodora was treated by other psychiatrists with first-generation antipsychotic medication (haloperidol, zuclopenthixol) for a long period with side effects such as dramatic chronic dystonia and dyskinesia. Dr. Georgila faced many side effects of the pharmacotherapy by Theodora and prescribed clozapine, and every 6 months botulinum toxin injection in order to reverse dystonia and dyskinesia. CBTp [33] was implemented by Dr. Rakitzi between September 2008 and January 2010 with 70 sessions, in which we focused on psychopathology and social skills training. Positive and negative symptoms, social skills, and functional outcomes were improved. She has begun to travel a lot with her mother, to build a better social relationship with a friend, and to have a better quality of life in her daily routine. She didn't focus anymore on delusions or voices.

The traumatic experience of sexual abuse from the psychiatrist was treated with cognitive interventions focused on changing the beliefs of danger, loss of control, weakness, and entrapment. The therapeutic relationships with two women (Dr. Georgila & Dr. Rakitzi) have contributed a lot to decreasing the impact of the sexual abuse from the first psychiatrist.

Theodora was diagnosed with breast cancer during 2010 and died in 2011 after metastases in lung and brain. She was very strong during the cancer therapies.

Theodora gave us her permission in 2009 to use her case study in publications. It was very important for her that young psychiatrists and psychologists learn appropriately to assist patients with schizophrenia successfully.

Theodora was confronted with many difficult disorders: sexual abuse, schizophrenia, treatment-resistant schizophrenia, and cancer. The death of Theodora was also very painful for us, and we are very grateful that we had the opportunity to help her finding new meaning in her life.

Anna is now 45 years old and suffers from treatment-resistant schizophrenia. Her parents made an appointment with Dr. Rakitzi 20 years ago, in 2004 because Anna couldn't sleep, was very anxious and suspicious and expressed religious delusions. She was very aggressive toward her parents because she believed that they represented the devil. Anna was in a fight between God and the devil, and she represented the God. She also heard the voices of the god. She also had also a suicidal plan, in case she didn't meet God. Furthermore, she participated in 15 sessions, in which I tried to refer her to a psychiatrist implementing psychoeducation and explaining her vulnerability without success.

I cooperated with the parents in order to schedule an involuntary hospitalization in cooperation with the Greek justice system. Anna was exceptionally aggressive toward others and herself.

She was hospitalized for 2 months in a psychiatric department, and afterward she was transferred to a short-stay psychiatric hostel for 6 months. The psychiatric and psychological treatment in the public mental health sector was very intensive, but she wasn't convinced about the importance of the therapy.

Dr. Rakitzi had the parents of Anna in treatment and coordinated with the mental health experts in the public mental health sector. Anna came back home after 8 months and denied following the pharmacotherapy (olanzapine 20 mg). She refused any cooperation with Dr. Rakitzi, but she gave her permission to utilize her case study in publications in order to prove that pharmacotherapy and psychotherapy are not compelling.

A second involuntary hospitalization was organized once again. She stayed 2 months at the hospital, and the psychiatrists proposed clozapine. Anna refused the pharmacotherapy and didn't want any psychotherapy, and the parents decided to keep her in a closed psychiatric division for chronic mental health disorders.

Stefanos is 35 years old. He has suffered from TRS since the age of 17 years old. He was treated for 2 years between 2015 and 2017 by Dr. Georgila. Dr. Georgila gave olanzapine 30 mg and anxiolytic drugs (benzodiazepines) with low improvement, and afterward clozapine 200 mg have been given. He dropped out of Dr. Georgila. He came back to Dr. Georgila in 2024, describing the following: He was under 10 ECT courses and pharmacotherapy with clozapine with no improvement and with worsening of his cognitive function, which was a big problem by the beginning of the disorder. His obsessive-compulsive symptoms were also worsening. Pharmacotherapy is continued with clozapine (350 mg) and amisulpride (1200 mg) with the intention to minimize amisulpride because of akathisia. Stefanos is being now prepared to participate in a combination of evidence-based treatments in the context of the RECOVERYTRSGR, as described in Chap. 4 of this book.

Below cases that presented showed great difficulty in cooperation:

George is 26 years old and is treated by a public psychiatric department. He takes injectable medicine every month (aripiprazole). He looked for psychotherapy and heard about RECOVERYTRSGR. Furthermore, he had an appointment with Dr. Georgila initially, where he was introduced to how his follow-up should be changed as well as the agent. George is treated every 6 months by the psychiatrist of the public hospital, which is not enough and evidence-based. Then he had a session with Dr. Rakitzi to start the evaluation with the psychometric tools and to make an introduction to our program.

He wanted to begin with a systematic psychiatric treatment and psychotherapy, but when he was confronted with our systematic model and treatment, he told us that he was not ready to participate. George possibly belongs to TRS and the agent doesn't help effectively. He doesn't sleep well, he is very suspicious, and he hears voices all day. During our two sessions, it was clear that his treatment in a public psychiatric department every 6 months is not enough to cope with TRS. George will think about it in the future before participating in our program.

Nikos is 45 years old and suffers 15 years from TRS. He lives alone in the city center and has no support. He is treated by a private psychiatrist every 3 months and takes an injectable agent (olanzapine) monthly. His psychiatrist does not encourage him to do psychotherapies, believing that only medication is effective. He describes persistent hallucinations and has persistent negative symptoms and multiple cognitive deficits. He asked for a session by Dr. Georgila and Dr. Rakitzi to get information about RECOVERYTRSGR. The condition for participation in the program is that pharmacotherapy and psychotherapy are offered by us. Nikos will think about it to participate on RECOVERYTRSGR in the future.

Kostas is 45 years old and recently lost his mother, who was taking care of him. His brother turned to us for treatment. Kostas stopped the medication; he was in an acute psychotic episode with intense suicidal ideation and planning. We recommended hospitalization for a few days and the resumption of our cooperation after hospitalization.

Psychotherapy with schizophrenia and treatment-resistant schizophrenia presents an interesting journey to many destinations. Some destinations bring happiness, harmony, and a new meaning in life, and some destinations lead to weakness, pessimism, and the belief of the Greek philosopher Socrates: one thing I know is that I know nothing!

All the above-presented case studies are touching stories, which permit us to send a central message: Clinical experience, psychotherapeutic training, and the implementation of evidence-based psychotherapies and interventions at the individual and group level lead to long-term positive results and to the improvement of the quality of life of patients with treatment-resistant schizophrenia and their families. The following conclusions can be drawn:

Suicidality is the primary goal of the therapy for treatment-resistant schizophrenia. Most of the patients seek help, when suicidality emerges and brings numerous issues to them and their families. If the family has good interpersonal relationships, then suicidality can be coped with systematic ambulant psychiatric treatment and psychotherapy. If patients are alone without home care, then hospitalization is exceptionally possible. Suicidality must be under control before we proceed with further interventions.

The side effects of polypharmacy ought to be treated as a priority because they can lead to awful adherence to pharmacotherapy. Clozapine presents an imperative agent for treatment-resistant schizophrenia. Psychiatrists are often confronted with unwanted side effects of clozapine, which implies that clozapine ought to be interrupted. The advance of the therapy of these people without clozapine is exceptionally troublesome because they have to deal with treatment-resistant cognitive dysfunctions and positive and negative symptoms, which are not treated so well with other agents. Psychiatrists should offer systematic psychiatric treatment and refer them to psychotherapy.

Patients with treatment-resistant schizophrenia are very suspicious, socially isolated and have decreased motivation for anything in their lives. An individual cognitive-behavioral therapy is indicated at the beginning, so that those people can feel safe and secure and can be educated step by step in the process of psychotherapy. A good therapeutic relationship can be created after 20–30 sessions, and the participation in group therapy afterward can be easier. Patients with treatment-resistant schizophrenia need more time to feel safe with mental health experts and other patients, as well as with the process of psychotherapy, especially when they are confronted with non-evidence-based psychiatric treatment and psychotherapies.

Psychiatric treatment, cognitive behavioral psychotherapy, and rehabilitation ought to focus on specific therapeutic goals, which are also evidence-based. The improvement of cognitive functions, positive and negative symptoms, and psychopathology leads long-term to enhancement of functional outcome and quality of life.

It is apparent that treatment-resistant schizophrenia needs a combination of evidence-based interventions. The psychiatric treatment ought to be combined with psychoeducation, cognitive behavioral psychotherapy, metacognitive therapies, and rehabilitation programs. The impact of the above long-term therapeutic process ought to be assessed long term. It is very important to work synchronically with the TRS patient and his/her family or partner.

The cooperation between mental health experts-psychiatrists and psychologists-presents an important condition in order to offer compelling long-term psychiatric treatment and psychotherapy. This cooperation works in favor of the patients and their families.

The sexual abuse of a patient with treatment-resistant schizophrenia by a mental health expert is the entryway to suicidality. It is one of the most unethical issues in our profession. This person should work through the trauma of treatment-resistant schizophrenia and the trauma of abuse from a mental health expert. This can be a long process. A therapeutic relationship with respect and limits in combination with evidence-based interventions for TRS is the most excellent way to heal both traumata. Cognitive interventions should be implemented to work with the trauma of sexual abuse in TRS. The exposure to trauma in TRS can be very dangerous and lead to a backslide.

The main condition for participating in RECOVERYTRSGR is to be treated by us.

When patients with TRS refer to us to participate in RECOVERYTRSGR, they have to adapt to our intensive treatment conditions. When patients, for example, are treated every 6 months, they have to begin the TRS therapy from a new perspective. This is not easy for them.

When patients with TRS are confronted with an acute psychotic episode with suicidal ideation and a plan that cannot be treated on an outpatient basis, then we recommend hospitalization and resuming our collaboration in the context of RECOVERYTRSGR afterward.

Evidence-based psychiatric treatment and psychotherapy are available for patients and their families. Today, we are very proud of our colleagues, who create new therapies and publish studies with respect to their efficacy and effectiveness. These new therapies are available to us and to patients with TRS and their families.

On the other hand, not all the patients can take after our vision. A few patients are very negative toward therapy. We ought to attempt to improve their motivation toward evidence-based therapies. But a few patients will never take after our vision!

Taken together, case studies from clinical practice were presented. All these individuals were confronted with many problems regarding psychopathology and pharmacotherapy. The implementation of the correct combination of evidence-based interventions in a long-term basis was the right choice for a new restart in life and a reintegration into society. Suicidality should be treated as a first priority. Mental health experts must always highlight the importance of evidence-based interventions.

3.7 Discussion

TRS represents a chronic mental health disorder associated with persistent positive and negative symptoms, persistent cognitive dysfunction, more hospitalizations and higher suicide rates, poor compliance with pharmacological and psychotherapeutic therapies, and reduced quality of life.

Today, we cannot pretend that TRS doesn't exist! On the other hand, it is also one of the mental health disorders linked to high suicide rates. The sooner this is recognized, the better for the individual's life and that of their family.

The therapeutic relationship with patients with TRS and their families presents a very interesting experience. It activates the resources of mental health experts in the long-term. It is a very creative context that enables us to be motivated for changes and new adaptations in life. When patients with TRS and their families are looking for a new mental health expert, we hear the same history: they have been hospitalized many times after severe relapses, they have poor adherence to pharmacotherapy, they have lost their trust in science, and they want to die by suicide.

It is also very common to have a secondary benefit from TRS: patients have all the attention of the family on them; they don't need to try a lot because family solves problems in cases where interfamily relations are good; and finally, hallucinations and delusions are present most of the time the best "friends" of them. They describe an addictive and symbiotic relationship with delusions and hallucinations. Therefore, we need evidence-based interventions to educate them to go from an addictive and symbiotic relationship with the positive symptoms to more autonomy via *coping with them, from isolation and depression as a consequence of negative symptoms to more action for life and from cognitive dysfunction to better concentration, memory, and problem-solving.*

So we need to give them enough time and space to express themselves and make with them a new commitment; we show them a new way of coping with their mental health disorder and be the protagonist of their own life. Their family is also desperate and has no hope for something better in the future. The family should be the part of the therapy and contribute to the many and important changes. If the family behaves competitively and doesn't cooperate with the mental health experts, we should focus only on our cooperation with the patients with TRS.

Transparency, professionalism and evidence-based interventions are the right ingredients for building a safe and secure therapeutic relationship. A transparent explanation regarding evidence-based pharmacotherapy, psychotherapy, and rehabilitation gives hope and motivates patients and their families for new dimensions in life.

The therapeutic relationship displays a motivational context that enables mental health experts to be assertive toward sufferers of TRS, so that they can change step-by-step problems that have a great negative impact on functional outcomes. This assertive context activates a dynamic interpersonal therapeutic relationship that gives life a new meaning in life. We go from suicidal crisis, loneliness, despair, weakness, confinement and stigma to hope, self-responsibility toward their own problems, cohesive relationships with mental health experts and the family, and finally, activation of their own resources to cope every hour, every day, every week, every month, and every year with TRS. This procedure gives life a new meaning.

The therapeutic goals should be transparent in the context of the therapeutic relationship. Side effects of pharmacotherapy and polypharmacy should be treated as a first priority. This situation decreases the possibility of suicidal risk and bad adherence to pharmacotherapy. The next step should be the treatment of positive and negative symptoms and cognitive dysfunctions, which has a positive impact on functional outcomes. It is well known from research studies that positive symptoms are independent, and their improvement leads to a better functional outcome. Negative symptoms are related to cognitive functions and vice versa, *and their improvement leads to a positive impact on the functional outcome.*

Today, we can build up an appropriate therapeutic plan regarding the combination of evidence-based interventions and treat all the therapeutic goals.

The majority of patients with TRS show treatment-resistant cognitive dysfunctions. Cognitive dysfunctions are categorized in neurocognitive dysfunctions (information processing speed, concentration, working memory, memory, problem-solving) and in social cognitive dysfunctions (Theory of mind, attribution, social perception, social knowledge). Neurocognitive and social cognitive dysfunctions are separable categories. It is clear that concentration, memory, problem-solving, and the way we interpret the social interactions (social cognition) must be functional in order to communicate, to have interpersonal relationships, to live autonomously, and to work!

People with TRS are often traumatized by difficulties that arise over many years. They often face a late diagnosis of TRS, multiple pharmacological treatment phenomena, and multiple uses of non-evidence-based medications as well as non-evidence-based psychotherapies, which do not improve symptoms, increasing the likelihood of suicidality and reducing quality of life.

This condition leads to a loss of hope and faith and a growing distrust of therapies and professionals. Mental health professionals should accept the above behaviors when initiating therapy and strive to gain the trust of these individuals in the context of evidence-based pharmacotherapy and psychotherapy. Psychoeducation, appropriate pharmacotherapy for TRS without polypharmacy, and long-term recovery-oriented psychotherapy are steps that strengthen a new therapeutic relationship characterized by trust, hope, mutual understanding, greater transparency and democracy, and respect for the human rights of people with TRS. Individuals with TRS need to understand the meaning of TRS, the difficulties that arise from it, and the importance of taking specific medications and undergoing recovery-oriented psychotherapy.

TRS should be diagnosed as soon as possible. When clozapine can be given without causing serious health problems, it should be the medication of first choice. When clozapine cannot be administered, there are other possible combinations of antipsychotic medication. No more than two agents should be given. Polypharmacy increases the possibility of more side effects, non-compliance, relapse and suicidal thoughts and behavior, frequent hospitalizations, and death in some cases.

At last clozapine is the only hope as already mentioned. We all should count the patient's benefits toward the disadvantages and we should manage our anxiety and doubts.

ECT can be an alternative after the failure of the appropriate pharmacotherapy, such as clozapine and other antipsychotic agents, in combination with evidence-based psychotherapy and rehabilitation. ECT should be the last choice for clinical psychiatrists and should be implemented by very experienced clinical psychiatrists. Our experience with TRS all these years showed that long-term pharmacotherapy with clozapine and other antipsychotic agents in the context of long-term psychotherapy is enough to reach a very good functional outcome. ECT can also be very traumatic for patients with TRS and their families, and it can destroy a therapeutic relationship. So being very careful with such a decision is the most important thing. Cost and benefits of ECT should always be considered. Sometimes it is better to be patient with the slow improvement of patients with TRS. When especially suicidal risk is under control, we can wait for progress.

Psychoeducation, CBTp, CR-T, rehabilitation programs, MCT, MERIT, cognitive behavioral family therapy, and recovery programs presenting evidence-based psychotherapies to TRS. Relapse prevention should always be included in evidence-based psychotherapy. Further studies on the efficacy and effectiveness of the above interventions for TRS are appropriate. Further research is needed on the effectiveness of evidence-based pharmacotherapy and psychotherapy in such a difficult diagnostic category, such as TRS.

When people with TRS are exposed to trauma, such as abuse, trauma exposure should not be implemented but should be worked more with cognitive interventions in the context of CBTp and CR-T. These interventions reduce patterns of vulnerability, weakness, loneliness, mistrust, and loss of control and increase positive beliefs about self, others, and the future, strengthening resilience.

MCT and MERIT may improve symptoms, cognitive function, and quality of life through a metacognitive perspective. An integrated rehabilitation program aimed at improving symptoms, cognitive function, social skills, and problem-solving can then promote social reintegration. Rehabilitation programs and cognitive behavioral family therapy can also promote social reintegration and a sense of safety in the world.

The comorbidity of TRS and severe personality disorder should be treated with special care. TRS with avoidant, dependent, obsessive-compulsive, schizotypal and narcissistic personality disorders can participate in an individual setting as well as in a group setting with other personality disorders without many obstacles. TRS with obsessive-compulsive disorder and obsessive-compulsive personality disorder displays a difficult case that takes longer to stabilize and to build an appropriate therapeutic relationship. On the other hand, it is possible to participate in a group therapy without many difficulties. These patients with TRS try every moment to have control over their situation, although TRS is the best example of losing control. TRS with borderline, histrionic, schizoid, and antisocial personality disorders have more problems in a group setting.

It is recommended to begin with those personality disorders with an individual cognitive behavioral therapy and try to carry on with group cognitive behavioral therapy and rehabilitation. If this is not possible, it is recommended to carry on with an individual cognitive behavioral therapy for schizophrenia and personality disorders.

Antisocial personality disorder doesn't respect others and their rights, and it shows criminal behavior many times. Schizoid prefers lonely activities; histrionic seeks always intensive attention; and borderline personality disorder shows unstable and impulsive behavior all the time. All these parameters decrease the possibility of remaining in a group psychotherapeutic setting.

Severe personality disorders should be treated according to the cognitive behavioral model of Beck [75]. *Interventions on the level of personality that focuses on the restructure of the main schemas of the personality disorder contribute to an increase in functional outcomes in the daily routine.*

On the other side, if TRS is being treated properly, this could also have a positive impact also on the personality disorder. TRS is the main diagnosis on which we should focus the therapy. Personality disorder should be treated after the stabilization of TRS.

The combination of TRS and borderline personality disorder antisocial, schizoid and histrionic personality disorder is one of the most difficult, according to clinical experience. An antisocial personality disorder doesn't accept the rules of society. These people destroy every interpersonal relationship and are dangerous, showing criminal behavior. A borderline personality disorder shows impulsive, unstable, and auto-destructive behavior. If this impulsive behavior is affected by the positive symptoms, such as hallucinations, this is a very critical situation. A schizoid prefers lonely activities, and this increases the possibility coming to a group therapy. A histrionic personality seeks for attention all the time! So, it is very important to have them in an individual setting of cognitive behavioral therapy and rehabilitation for schizophrenia and personality disorders, and afterward to propose that they participate in a group setting with other members having the same problems, such as TRS and borderline, antisocial, schizoid, and histrionic personality disorder.

People with TRS exhibit treatment-resistant positive and negative symptoms, cognitive dysfunction as well as high suicidality. This means that long-term recovery-oriented pharmacotherapy and psychotherapy should be applied. It is known that people with TRS need more time to improve their quality of life.

The presented case studies showed the complexity and difficulties as well as the chances of TRS treatment. Suicidality is the first priority for these patients. The sooner the antisuicidal plan is activated the better for the sufferers from TRS. Negative experiences regarding side effects with agents, polypharmacy or not-necessary ECT, and non-evidence-based psychotherapy and rehabilitation should be discussed openly without stereotypes and avoidant strategies from mental health experts. RECOVERYTRSGR, a recovery-oriented program that is discussed in Chap. 4, offers a very intensive treatment with many sessions. Patients with TRS, who come to participate in it, often have other experiences with other colleagues. They have their psychiatric treatment every 6 months without participating in psychotherapy or the psychiatrist doesn't encourage them to participate in an intensive integrative treatment in which psychiatric treatment is combined with long-term evidence-based psychotherapy.

A central message should be sent: A democratic society is responsible for protecting vulnerable people by showing ways of being assertive toward their rights or the violation of their rights. This context will help sufferers from TRS and their families to build a new and stable therapeutic relationship with the mental health experts that will lead to a new restart of the treatment. A long-term combination of evidence-based interventions regarding pharmacotherapy, psychotherapy, and rehabilitation is the only way to a new restart in life. The experience of physical, psychological, and sexual abuse by patients with TRS makes the therapy more difficult and our responsibility toward them bigger. Especially, the abuse from mental health experts, as it was described in one of our cases, is the most difficult situation for all of us. It is also one of the most unethical behavior in our profession. Exposure to trauma is not recommended.

All the evidence-based interventions for TRS (psychoeducation, CBT, CR-T, rehabilitation) should be implemented so that the schemas of loss of control, weakness, vulnerability, and abandonment as a consequence of the trauma can be restructured. A safe and structured therapeutic relationship that activates resources and gives life a new meaning is the best balance and answer toward an abusive relationship that led to trauma.

Case studies showed that evidence-based interventions for TRS are nowadays available. As mental health experts, we ought to update our education regarding these interventions and to make these modern treatments known to the community through books, journal papers, participation in conferences, workshops, and other social media. Private and public mental health departments should evaluate to determine whether evidence-based interventions are being offered and how effective and efficacious their implementation is.

Living with TRS and a chronic mental health disorder means the activation of a grief process, which should be expressed. Denial, anger, bargaining, depression, and acceptance are the five stages of the grief process that are expressed via *psychotic symptoms regarding the co-existence of a chronic mental health disorder.*

Clinical psychiatrists and clinical psychologists should be very careful with those phases that are associated with high suicidal risk and bad adherence to pharmacotherapy.

The patients with TRS and their families suffer from an intensive grief process throughout their lives. It takes time to accept a long-term vulnerability with negative consequences for your whole life.

Individual psychiatric treatment and individual sessions of cognitive behavioral psychotherapy are essential dealing with the grief process. Family sessions are also recommended if all the family members suffer at the same time from active grief. It is very difficult to fight with such a disorder with so many consequences on emotional, behavioral, and cognitive levels and on quality of life. Patients with TRS and their families should have the opportunity to express their grief in a safe and structured psychotherapeutic setting. This confrontation with the grief leads to a post-psychotic depression in short term but prepares the road to a long term and new restart in life. The sooner the grief process is being treated, the better for the sufferers from TRS.

Patients with TRS understand that this disorder has a strong biological basis and, in combination with psychological vulnerability, can lead to a relapse or a psychotic episode. In other words, patients with TRS understand that pharmacotherapy is the main therapy, and without it, a relapse is very possible. The participation on a combination of evidence-based psychotherapy and rehabilitation is the next step.

The long-term participation in evidence-based treatments transforms the grief process into an action for life, for improvement and for a new reintegration into society and a new restart in life. The grief process can be activated in any phases of the lives of people with TRS and their families. Long-term action against TRS through evidence-based interventions is the best way to express this grief.

The long-term grief of TRS sufferers and their families can cause depression and should be an important therapeutic goal in the context of CBT aiming to the relief from grief and acceptance of the illness.

The combination of different psychotherapies at multiple levels, such as individual therapy, group therapy, and family therapy with the possibility of repeating after a year or two, is the appropriate way to address treatment resistance in schizophrenia. The menu of available interventions is broad enough to incorporate different evidence-based psychotherapies. *Recovery-oriented interventions lead patients with TRS and their families from long-term grief process to action for step-by step improvement in the daily routine and to action for gaining more goals in life.*

Recovery as an outcome and recovery as a process must be two different perspectives, coexisting with each other, and should be considered when evaluating the outcomes of reintegrating into society for people with TRS.

What should be done in the future? Effective pharmacotherapy without polypharmacy or side effects is essential for TRS. The combination of evidence-based interventions in the context of CBT and rehabilitation with the possibility of repeating psychotherapy constitutes the treatment of choice for TRS, which should be the primary focus of the protocol's future research.

The long-term intervention, in which treatments will be combined, will lead to stable ambulant treatment with stable reference persons-therapists. Fixed ambulant places build a home and a family! Whatever bad happens, these frameworks are there to absorb crises and pave the way for recovery.

The long-term therapeutic relationship will go through difficult and pleasant moments. The main denominator of all is communication around issues that make everyday life difficult and increase dysfunctional behavior. The compass of the therapeutic relationship is the empirically documented interventions and how these are applied at the appropriate level.

Mental health professionals must be dedicated to their work in order to do their best to accompany patients with TRS and their families with dignity, professionalism, and efficiency. Finally, this long-term therapeutic relationship is a very beautiful journey. It is an honor for experts to have this role in the lives of our vulnerable fellow citizens.

Mental health experts must never forget what TRS means: there are specific pharmacotherapies that are recommended, psychotherapy must be long term, and combine various interventions and at the same time, must give the possibility of repeating them.

In summary, TRS presents a challenge for mental health experts and should be diagnosed as soon as possible. Treatment-resistant positive and negative symptoms, as well as cognitive dysfunctions, are at the forefront. This situation is associated with high suicidal risk. The therapeutic relationship should be a motivational context that leads to changes step by step, enhancing the personal responsibility for their own problems. Polypharmacy presents an ineffective strategy. Today, evidence-based pharmacotherapy for TRS is available to us. Clozapine, with or without a combination with other antipsychotic agents, should be the first choice. Evidence-based cognitive behavioral psychotherapy and rehabilitation should be combined in long term with pharmacotherapy. Case studies displayed the importance of evidence-based interventions. ECT must not be an easy alternative.

It can be very traumatic for the patients with TRS and their families, and it can destroy the therapeutic relationship. According to our experience, long-term evidence-based treatment-pharmacotherapy, and cognitive behavioral psychotherapy and rehabilitation-without ECT can solve the problems of TRS. TRS and comorbid severe personality disorders need special attention. Finally, the grief process regarding the confrontation with a chronic mental health disorder should be treated properly.

3.8 Conclusions

Schizophrenia and TRS are serious chronic mental health disorders. TRS is a separate category. It is associated with suicidal risk. Evidence-based, recovery-oriented pharmacotherapy and psychotherapy are the first-choice treatments. Relapse prevention should also be an important part of treatment. Case studies have demonstrated the importance of a recovery-oriented treatment approach. Finally, the authors' description of an ongoing research process demonstrates the importance of bridging the gap between research and clinical practice.

Revision Questions

1. Please define schizophrenia.
2. Please define TRS.
3. Is TRS a distinct category?
4. Why is TRS difficult?
5. Evidence-based pharmacotherapy for TRS.
6. Evidence-based psychotherapy for TRS.
7. What should be done to improve evidence-based pharmacotherapy and psychotherapy in TRS?
8. Please describe and clarify the recovery as an outcome and the recovery as a process in TRS.
9. Please describe the metacognitive model of relapse prevention in TRS.
10. Which elements regarding TRS should be the focus of research in the future?

Competing Interests The authors have no conflicts of interest to declare that are relevant to the content of this chapter.

Ethical Approval Our case studies follow the ethical standards of the 1964 Declaration of Helsinki and its amendments. Informed consent to publish was obtained from individual participants.

The authors organize an annual seminar about the evidence-based treatments of CBT and rehabilitation for treatment-resistant schizophrenia for clinical psychologists, clinical psychiatrists, and cognitive-behavioral psychotherapists. The authors also provide training in Integrated Psychological Therapy (Schizophrenia) annually to Greek clinical psychologists, psychiatrists, and cognitive-behavioral psychotherapists in Greece. For more information, please visit https://www.linkedin.com/in/stavroula-rakitzi-0b512b45/, http://orcid.org/0000-0002-5231-6619 (Stavroula Rakitzi), https://gr.linkedin.com/in/polyxeni-georgila-940b521a7, http://orcid.org/0000-0003-3137-506x (Polyxeni Georgila) or email srakitzi@gmail.com.

References

1. Howes OD, Thase ME, Pillinger T. Treatment resistance in psychiatry: state of the art and new directions. Mol Psychiatry. 2022;27:58–72. https://doi.org/10.1038/s41380-021-01200-3.
2. Millgate E, Hide O, Lawrie SM, Murray RM, MacCabe JH, Kravariti E. Neuropsychological differences between treatment resistant and treatment responsive schizophrenia: a meta-analysis. Psychol Med. 2022;52:1–13. https://doi.org/10.1017/S0033291721004128.
3. Potkin SG, Kane JM, Correll CU, Lindenmayer JP, Agid O, Marder SR, Olfson M, Howes OD. The neurobiology of treatment-resistant schizophrenia: paths to antipsychotic resistance and a roadmap for future research. NPJ Schizophr. 2020;6:1. https://doi.org/10.1038/s41537-019-0090-z.
4. Correll CU, Howes OD. Treatment-resistant schizophrenia: definitions, predictors and therapy options. J Clin Psychiatry. 2022;82(5). https://doi.org/10.4088/CPMY20096AH1C.
5. Keepers GA, Fochtmann LJ, Anzia JM, Benjamin S, Lyness JM, Mojtabai R, Servis M, Walaszeck A, Buckley P, Lenzenweger MF, Young AS, Degenhardt A, Hong SH. The American

Psychiatric Association practice guideline for the treatment of patients with schizophrenia. Am J Psychiatry. 2020;177:9. ajp.psychiatryonline.org
6. Galderisi S, Kaiser S, Bitter I, Nordentoft M, Mucci A, Sabé M, Giordano GM, Nielsen MØ, Glenthøj LB, Dollfus S, Pezella P, Falkai P, Dollfus S, Gaebel W. EPA guidance on treatment of negative symptoms in schizophrenia. Eur Psychiatry. 2021;64(1):e21. https://doi.org/10.1192/j.eurpsy.2021.13.
7. Vita A, Gaebel W, Mucci A, Sachs G, Barlati S, Giordano GM, Nibbio G, Nordentoft M, Wykes T, Galderisi S. European Psychiatric Association Guidance on treatment of cognitive impairment in schizophrenia. Eur Psychiatry. 2022;65(1):e57. https://doi.org/10.1192/j.eurpsy.2022.2315.
8. Gaebel W, Grossimlinghaus I, Kerst A, Cohen Y, Hinsche-Böckenholt A, Johnson B, Muck D, Petrea I, Rössler W, Thornicroft G, Zielasek J. European Psychiatric Association (EPA) guidance on the quality of eMental health interventions in the treatment of psychotic disorders. Eur Arch Psychiatry Clin Neurosci. 2016;266:125–37. https://doi.org/10.1007/s00406-016-0677-6.
9. Correll CU, Brevig T, Brain C. Exploration of treatment resistant schizophrenia subtypes based on a survey of 204 US Psychiatrists. Neuropsychiatr Dis Treat. 2019;15:3461–73. https://doi.org/10.2147/NDT.S234813.
10. Gillespie AM, Samanaite R, Mill J, Egerton A, MacCabe JH. Is treatment-resistant schizophrenia categorically distinct from treatment-responsive schizophrenia? A systematic review. BMC Psychiatry. 2017;17:12. https://doi.org/10.1186/s12888-016-1177-y.
11. Ali SA, Mathur N, Malhotra AK, Braga RJ. Electroconvulsive therapy and schizophrenia: a systematic review. Mol Neuropsych. 2019;5:75–83. https://doi.org/10.1159/000497376.
12. Silvo J, Moto J, Azevedo P. Electoconvulsive therapy in schizophrenia-where do we stand? Eur Psych. 2016;33:S262–3. https://doi.org/10.1016/j.eurpsy.2016.01.671.
13. Petrides G, Malur C, Braga RJ, Bailine SH, Schooler NR, Malhotra AK, Kane JM, Sanghani S, et al. Electroconvulsive therapy Augmentation in clozapine-resistant schizophrenia: a prospective randomized study. Am J Psychiatry. 2015;172:52–8. https://doi.org/10.1176/appi.ajp.201413060787.
14. Keepers GA, Fochtmann LJ, Anzia JM, Benjamin S, Lyness JM, Mojtabai R, Servis M, Walaszeck A, Buckley P, Lenzenweger MF, Young AS, Degenhardt A, Hong SH. The American Psychiatric Association. Practice guideline for the treatment of patients with schizophrenia. American Psychiatric Association; 2021.
15. American Psychiatric Association. Diagnostic and statistical manual of mental disorders. DSM 5-TR. Washington, DC: American Psychiatric Publishing; 2022.
16. Kumari S, Malik M, Florival C, Manalai P, Sonje S. An assessment of five (PANSS, SAPS, SANS, NSA-16, CGI-SCH) commonly used symptoms ratings scales in schizophrenia and comparison to newer scales (CAINS, BNSS). J Addict Res Ther. 2017;8(3):324. https://doi.org/10.4172/2155-6105.1000324.
17. Nuecterlein KH, Green MF. MATRICS consensus cognitive battery. Los Angeles: MATRICS Assessment Inc.; 2006.
18. Mørup MF, Kymmes SM, Aström DQ. A modeling approach to estimate the prevalence of treatment resistant schizophrenia. PLoS One. 2020;15(6):e0234121. https://doi.org/10.1371/journal.pone.0234121.
19. Kadra-Scalzo G, de Freitas DF, Agbedjro D, Francis E, Ridler I, Pritchard M, Shetty H, Segev A, Casetta C, Smart SE, Morris A, Downs J. A predictor model of treatment resistance in schizophrenia using data from electronic health records. PLoS ONE. 2022;17(9):e0274864. https://doi.org/10.1371/journal.pone.0274864.
20. Huhn M, Nikolakopoulou A, Schneider-Thoma J, Krause M, Samara M, Peter N, Leucht S, et al. Comparative efficacy and tolerability of 32 oral antipsychotics for the acute treatment of adults with multi-episode schizophrenia: a systematic review and network meta analysis. Lancet. 2019;394:939–51. https://doi.org/10.1016/S0140-6736(19)31135-3.

21. Leucht S, Cipriani A, Spineli L, Mavridis D, Őrey D, Richter F, Davis JM, et al. Comparative efficacy and tolerability of 15 antipsychotic drugs in schizophrenia: a multiple-treatments meta-analysis. Lancet. 2013;382(9896):951–62. https://doi.org/10.1016/S0140-6736(13)60733-3.
22. Taipale H, Mehtälä J, Tanskanen A, Tiihonen J. Comparative effectiveness of antipsychotics drugs for rehospitalization in schizophrenia. A Nationwide study with 20 year follow up. Schizophr Bull. 2018;44(6):1381–7. https://doi.org/10.1093/schbul/sbx176.
23. Tandon R. Antipsychotics in the treatment of schizophrenia: an overview. J Clin Psychiatry. 2018;72(Suppl. 1). https://doi.org/10.4088/JCP.10075su1.01.
24. Fernández-Sotos P, Navarro E, Torio I, Dompablo M, Fernández-Caballero A, Rodriguez-Jimenez R. Pharmacological interventions in social cognition deficits: a systematic mapping review. Psychiatry Res. 2018;270:57–67. https://doi.org/10.1016/j.psychres.2018.09.012.
25. Kucharksa-Pietura K, Mortimer A. Can antipsychotics improve social cognition in patients with schizophrenia? CNS Drugs. 2013;27:335–43. https://doi.org/10.1007/2Fs40263-013-0047-0.
26. Correll CU, Agid O, Crespo-Facorro B, de Bartolomeis A, Fagiolini A, Seppala N, Howes OD. A guideline and checklist for initiating and managing clozapine treatment in patients with treatment-resistant schizophrenia. CNS Drugs. 2022;36:659–79. https://doi.org/10.1007/s40263-022-00932-2.
27. Citrome L. Treatment-refractory schizophrenia: what is it and what has been done about it? Neuropsychiatry. 2011;1(4):325–47. https://doi.org/10.2217/npy.11.35.
28. Wagner E, Siafis S, Fernando P, Falkai P, Honer WG, Röh A, Siskind D, Leucht S, Hasan A. Efficacy and safety of clozapine in psychotic disorders. A systematic quantitative meta-review. Transl Psychiatry. 2021;11:487. https://doi.org/10.1038/s41398-021-01613-2.
29. De Bartolomeis A, Ciccarelli M, Vellucci L, Formaro M, Iasevoli F, Barone A. Update on novel antipsychotics and pharmacological strategies for treatment-resistant schizophrenia. Expert Opin Pharmacother. 2022;23(18):2035–52.
30. Samara MT, Dold M, Gianatsi M, Nikolakopoulou A, Helfer B, Salanti G, Leucht S. Efficacy, acceptability and tolerability of antipsychotics in treatment-resistant schizophrenia. A network meta-analysis. JAMA Psych. 2016;73(3):199–210. https://doi.org/10.1001/jamapsychiatry.2015.2955.
31. Pandey A, Kalita KN. Treatment-resistant schizophrenia: how far have we traveled? Front Psych. 2022;(13):994425. https://doi.org/10.3389/fpsyt.2022.994425.
32. Zubin J, Spring BJ. Vulnerability—a new view of schizophrenia. J Abnorm Psychol. 1977;86:103–26.
33. Beck AT, Rector NA, Stolar N, Grant P. Schizophrenia. Cognitive theory, research and therapy. New York: The Guilford Press; 2009.
34. Beck AT, Grant P, Inverso E, Brinen AP, Perivoliotis D. Recovery oriented cognitive therapy for serious mental health conditions. New York: The Guilford Press; 2021.
35. Grant PM, Bredemeier K, Beck AT. Six month follow up of recovery-oriented cognitive therapy for low functioning individuals with schizophrenia. Psychiatr Serv. 2017;68(10):997–1002.
36. Moritz S, Menon M, Balzan R, Woodward TS. Metacognitive training for psychosis (MCT): past, present and future. Europ Archiv Psychiat Clin Neurosci. 2022. https://doi.org/10.1007/s00406-022-01394-9.
37. Penney D, Sauvé G, Mendelson D, Thibaudeau E, Moritz S, Lepage M. Immediate and sustained outcomes and moderators associated with metacognitive training for psychosis. A systematic review and meta-analysis. JAMA Psychiat. https://doi.org/10.1001/jamapsychiatry.2022.0277.
38. Veckenstedt R, Scheunemann J. Metakognitives training für Patientinnen mit Psychose in Gruppen- und Einzelsetting. Psychotherapeut J. 2023;2023(3):255–60.
39. Lysaker P, Klion R. Recovery, meaning-making and severe mental illness: a comprehensive guide to metacognitive reflection and insight therapy. New York: Routledge; 2017.
40. Lysaker PH, Gagen E, Klion R, Zalzala A, Vohs J, Faith LA, Leonhardt B, Hamm J, Hasson-Ohayson I. Metacognitive reflection and insight therapy: a recovery-oriented treatment approach for psychosis. Psychol Res Behav Manag. 2020;13:331–41. https://doi.org/10.2147/PRBM.S198628.

41. Rakitzi S, Georgila P, Becker-Woitag AP. The recovery process for individuals with schizophrenia in the context of evidence-based psychotherapy and rehabilitation. Eur Psychol. 2021;26(2):96–111. https://doi.org/10.1027/1016-9040/a000400.
42. Roder V, Medalia A, editors. Neurocognition and social cognition in schizophrenia patients. Basic concepts and treatment. Basel: Karger; 2010.
43. Rakitzi S, Georgila P, Efthimiou K, Müller DR. Efficacy and feasibility of the Integrated Psychological Therapy for outpatients with schizophrenia in Greece: final results of a RCT. Psychiatry Res. 2016;242:137–43. https://doi.org/10.1016/j.psychres.2016.05.039.
44. Rakitzi S, Georgila P. Integrated Psychological Therapy and treatment resistant schizophrenia: initial findings. Psychiatry. 2019;82(4):354–67. https://doi.org/10.1080/00332747.2019.1616658.
45. Twamley EW, Savla GN, Zurhellen CH, Heaton RK, Jeste DV. Development and pilot testing of a novel compensatory cognitive training intervention for people with psychosis. Am J Psychiatr Rehabil. 2008;11:144–63.
46. Roder V, Mueller DR, Schmidt SJ. Effectiveness of Integrated Psychological Therapy (IPT) for schizophrenia patients. Schizophr Bull. 2011;37(Suppl. 2):71–9. https://doi.org/10.1093/schbul/sbr072.
47. Mueller DH, Schmidt SJ, Roder V. Integrated Psychological Therapy. Effectiveness in schizophrenia inpatient settings related to patients age. Am J Geriatr Psychiatry. 2013;21(3):231–41. https://doi.org/10.1016/j.jagp.2012.12.011.
48. Mueller DR, Schmidt SJ, Roder V. One year randomized controlled trial and follow up of Integrated Neurocognitive Therapy for schizophrenia outpatients. Schizophr Bull. 2015;41(3):604–16. https://doi.org/10.1093/schbul/sbu223.
49. Rakitzi S. Grundlagen evidenzbasierter Rehabilitation von Schizophrenieerkrankten. Basics of evidence-based Rehabilitation in individuals with schizophrenia. Doctoral thesis. Universität Koblenz-Landau, Campus Landau, Universitätsbibliothek; 2020.
50. Palumbo D, Mucci A, Giordano GM, Piegari G, Aiello C, Pietrafesa D, Annarumma N, Chieffi M, Cella M, Galderisi S. The efficacy, feasibility and acceptability of a remotely accessible use of CIRCuiTs. A computerized cognitive remediation therapy program for schizophrenia: a pilot study. Neuropsych Diseas Treat. 2019;15:3103–13. https://doi.org/10.2147/NDT.S221690.
51. Mueser KT, Meyer PS, Penn DL, Clancy R, Clancy DM, Salyers MP. The illness management and recovery program: rationale, development and preliminary findings. Schizophr Bull. 2006;(Suppl. 1):32–43. https://doi.org/10.1093/schbul/sbl022.
52. Hofmann SG, Asnaani A, Vonk IJJ, Sawyer AT, Fang A. The efficacy of cognitive behavioral therapy: a review of meta-analyses. Cogn Ther Res. 2012;36(5):427–40. https://doi.org/10.1007/s10608-012-9476-1.
53. Falloon IRH, Roncone R, Held T, Coverdale JH, Laidlaw TM. An international overview of family interventions: developing effective treatment strategies and measuring their benefits for patients, carers, and communities. In: Lefley HP, Johnson DL, editors. Family interventions in mental illness: international perspectives. Praeger Publishers/Greenwood Publishing Group; 2002. p. 3–23.
54. Falloon IRH. Behavioral family therapy. In: Gurman AS, Kniskern DP, editors. Handbook of family therapy, vol. 2. Brunner/Mazel; 1991. p. 65–95.
55. Schmidt SJ, Mueller DR, Roder V. Social cognition as a mediator between neurocognition and functional outcome in schizophrenia: empirical review and new results by structural equation modelling. Schizophr Bull. 2011;37(2):41–54.
56. Killapsy H, Craig T, Dark F, Harvey C, Medalia A. Editorial: design and implementation of rehabilitation interventions for people with complex psychosis. Front Psych. 2021;12:698432. https://doi.org/10.3389/fpsyt.2021.698432.
57. Morrison AP, Law H, Carter L, Sellers R, Emsley P, Pyle M, et al. antipsychotic drug versus cognitive behavioral therapy versus a combination of both in people with psychosis: a randomized controlled pilot and feasibility study. Lancet Psychiatry. 2018;5(5):411–23. https://doi.org/10.1016/S2215-0366(18)30096-8.

58. Klingberg S, Wölwer W, Engel C, Wittorf A, Herrlich J, Meisner C, et al. Negative symptoms of schizophrenia as primary target of cognitive behavioral therapy: results of randomized Clinical TONES study. Schizophr Bull. 2011;(Suppl. 2):98–110.
59. Mehl S, Werner D, Lincoln T. Corrigendum: does cognitive behaviour for psychosis (CBTp) show a sustainable effect on delusions? A meta-analysis. Front Psychol. 2019;10:1868. https://doi.org/10.3389/fpsyg.2019.01868.
60. Morin L, Franck N. Rehabilitation interventions to promote recovery from schizophrenia. A systematic review. Front Psych. 2017;8:100. https://doi.org/10.3389/fpsyt.2017.00100.
61. Pfammatter M, Junghan UM, Brenner HD. Efficacy of psychological therapy in schizophrenia: conclusions of meta-analyses. Schizophr Bull. 2006;32:64–80. https://doi.org/10.1093/2Fschbul/2Fsbl030.
62. Miller WR, Rollnick S. Motivational interviewing: preparing people for change. New York: The Guilford Press; 2002.
63. Rakitzi S. Clinical psychology and cognitive behavioral psychotherapy. Recovery in mental health. Cham, Switzerland: Springer; 2023.
64. Granholm E, Twamley EW, Mahmood Z, Keller AV, Lykins HC, Parrish EM, Thomas ML, Perivoliotis D, Holden JL. Integrated cognitive behavioral social skills training and compensatory cognitive training for negative symptoms of psychosis: effects in a pilot randomized controlled trial. Schizophr Bull. 2022;48(2):359–70.
65. Citrome L. Handbook of treatment-resistant schizophrenia. Springer Healthcare Tarporley; 2013. https://doi.org/10.1007/978-1-908517-88-3.
66. Rakitzi S, Georgila P. The combination of pharmacotherapy, IPT and MCT in individuals with schizophrenia. Clinical Trial Registration (NCT 05623228); 2022.
67. Kosmidou M, Vlahou X. Greek verbal memory test. Athens: Parisianos; 2010.
68. Kay SR, Fiszbein A, Opler LA. The positive and negative syndrome scale (PANSS) for schizophrenia. Schizopr Bull. 1987;13(2):261–76.
69. Haddock G, McCarron J, Tarrier N, Faragher EB. Scales to measure dimensions of hallucinations and delusions: the psychotic symptom rating scales (PSYRATS). Psychol Med. 1999;29(4):879–89.
70. World Health Organization. International classification of functioning, disability and health (ICF). Geneva: World Health Organization; 2001.
71. Koumpouros Y, Papageorgiou E, Sakellari E, et al. Adaptation and psychometric properties' evaluation of the Greek version of WHODAS 2.0. Pilot application in Greek elderly population. Health Serv Outcomes Res Methodol. 2018;18(1):63–74. https://doi.org/10.1007/s10742-017-0176-x.
72. Hancock N, Scanlan JN, Bundy AC, Honey A. Recovery Assessment Scale-Domains & Stages (RAS-DS) manual-version 3. Sydney: University of Sydney; 2019.
73. Hancock N, the University of Sydney, Rakitzi S. Katoudi S. Recovery Assessment Scale-Domains & Stages (RAS-DS). The Greek version; 2023.
74. Aster M, Neubauer M, Horn R. Wechsler-Intelligenztest für Erwachsene WIE. Frankfurt: Harcourt Test Services; 2006.
75. Beck AT, Freeman A, Davis DD, Associates. Cognitive therapy of personality disorders. 2nd ed. New York: The Guilford Press; 2004.

A New Recovery-Oriented Treatment Model for Treatment-Resistant Schizophrenia. A Greek Model (RECOVERYTRSGR)

4

Learning Objectives

1. A new recovery-oriented pharmacotherapy for TRS.
2. A new recovery-oriented psychotherapy for TRS.
3. Advantages and disadvantages of this new model.

4.1 Introduction

The long clinical experience and collaboration of Dr. S. Rakitzi and Dr. P. Georgila came up with the idea of developing a recovery-focused therapy model for TRS. More than 30% of people with schizophrenia have TRS, which is associated with high suicide rates, more cognitive dysfunction, more hospitalizations, and frequent relapses. All of these factors have contributed to the development of a new recovery-oriented model.

The Greek health system has many structural problems. The mental health system in Greece is multidimensional; various psychotherapies are applied, but without evaluating their effectiveness. Patients with TRS go from hospital to hospital without having done systematic therapeutic work that will deal with the problem at its root. Thus, there was born a need to create a structured and effective model for TRS that will provide solutions to the chronic problems of patients and their families.

Additionally, the disappointment of patients with TRS, their long-term grief, their frustration, and the continued suicidal crisis have motivated us to focus on the development of a structured and evidence-based program for TRS, in which patients and their families are included in a collaborative context.

Long-term participation in such a program can lead sufferers of TRS to work systematically with problems and to find a new meaning in life with more resilience and hope.

S. Rakitzi, P. Georgila, *Treatment-Resistant Schizophrenia*,
https://doi.org/10.1007/978-3-031-64623-2_4

There are well-known etiological models of schizophrenia that were considered in our model.

The underlying pathophysiology of schizophrenia is dysfunction of the *dopaminergic, glutamatergic, serotonergic, and gamma-aminobutyric acid signaling systems* [1].

Zubin and Spring's [2] *vulnerability-stress model* describes the relationship between vulnerability and stress. High vulnerability in stressful situations can lead to psychotic episodes. Vulnerability factors may include discontinuation of drug therapy, strong feelings of family members toward the person with TRS, alcohol and substance abuse, or lack of sleep. Stress is something that is always present, for example, due to financial problems, unemployment, or the death of a loved one. When vulnerability is controlled or reduced, individuals become more capable of coping with stress.

The *Green and Nuchterlein model* [3] presents a strong relationship between neurocognition and negative symptoms, as well as between neurocognition and functional outcome. Neurocognitive dysfunction has a negative impact on functional outcomes [3]. Social cognition mediates the association between neurocognition and functional outcomes [3, 4].

Brenner's two vicious cycle model [5] describes the negative impact of cognitive vulnerability on social competence. Dysfunction of simple cognitive variables, such as the ability to concentrate, has a negative impact on more complex cognitive dysfunctions, such as impaired memory and executive function. These lead to dysfunction of social skills, increasing stress, and cognitive vulnerability, and thus further cognitive dysfunction.

Psychometric tests, such as the Matrics Consensus Cognitive Battery (MCCB) [6] for MCCB cognitive functions, Positive and Negative Syndrome Scale (PANSS) [7, 8], WHODAS 2 0 [9, 10] for disability and functional capacity, and the Recovery Assessment Scale-Domains and Stages (RAS-DS) [11, 12] offer valid and reliable tests, and they should be performed before, after treatment, and at follow-up 6 months. WAIS [13] should be used before treatment to show the burden of cognitive dysfunction and intellectual ability, and it is repeatable after 1 year. An intelligence quotient (IQ) $\geq$ 80 is a necessary condition to participate in our recovery model for TRS. Selection criteria: *Inclusion criteria:* age 18–65, IQ $\geq$ 80, diagnosis TRS. *Exclusion criteria:* Substance abuse and head injury. If substance abuse is successfully treated, the participant will be accepted into our program.

Our clinical experience with TRS has shown us the path to effective therapy for these people: *long-term recovery-oriented* pharmacotherapy and psychotherapy, with the possibility of *repeating* the treatment procedure. Individuals with TRS need more time to reset after negative experiences and build trust in the scientific community.

Well-known and evidence-based psychological therapies in individual and group settings, such as CBTp [14], CR-T [15], IPT [16, 17], and MCT [18, 19] are included and recommended because of their effectiveness and efficacy for people with schizophrenia and their international recognition in the scientific community. We are very grateful to the creators of the above therapies, such as Dr. A. Beck and his colleagues, Professor. H. D. Brenner, Professor. V. Roder and their colleagues, as well as Prof. S. Moritz and his colleagues, have made these treatments available to the scientific community. Finally, our proposal for implementing these psychotherapies in RECOVERYTRSGR (Fig. 4.1) presents the results of our clinical experience with them over the years [20] and our recognition of their usefulness and effectiveness in clinical practice.

There are three perspectives that play a central role in our model (RECOVERYTRSGR) (Fig. 4.1): The cognitive perspective, which focuses on our cognition (thoughts, beliefs, and schema), the metacognitive perspective, which is awareness of my thoughts, beliefs, and schema (thoughts about cognitions), and the recovery perspective, which focuses on recovery as an outcome or objective recovery (assessment of mental health from experts through psychometric tests), and recovery as a process or subjective recovery (the perspective of the person suffering from TRS and its family).

Our recovery-oriented therapy (RECOVERYTRSGR) (Fig. 4.1) consists of three phases: introduction, recovery-oriented therapy, and epilogue. The second phase includes a combination of evidence-based pharmacotherapy, cognitive-behavioral psychotherapy, and rehabilitation. Known and evidence-based psychotherapies are incorporated first in the context of individual therapy (cognitive phase) and second in the context of group therapy (rehabilitation and metacognitive phases). RECOVERYTRSGR (Fig. 4.1) contributes to the balance of neurotransmitters responsible for schizophrenia, improving insight by symptoms, cognitive function, social skills, and problem-solving, restructuring cognitive distortions related to delusions and hallucinations, improving family communication, and improving functional outcomes and recovery.

RECOVERYTRSGR (Fig. 4.1) aims to be implemented in the coming years in Greece and other countries and help as many people with TRS as possible.

In sum, the problems in the Greek health system as well as the problems with patients with TRS have motivated us to develop a structured and evidence-based recovery-oriented program. Our model is based on specific etiological models that are considered in our model. Inclusion and exclusion criteria for patients with TRS and the psychometric tests that can be used are described. RECOVERYTRSGR consists of three phases: introduction, recovery-oriented therapy, and epilogue. Evidence-based pharmacotherapy and psychotherapy are being offered. Finally, three perspectives—the cognitive, the metacognitive, and the recovery perspective—play an important role.

A. Introductory phase (3 months) (20 sessions)
Psychometric evaluation regarding intelligence, cognitive functions, symptoms, social skills and problem-solving, functional outcome and recovery before the intervention (recovery as an outcome).

1. Month: (8 sessions) two individual sessions of one hour per week, one session with the clinical psychiatrist and one session with the clinical psychologist and cognitive behavioral psychotherapist. Build of therapeutic relationship, psycho-education, motivational interviewing, negative past experiences with treatments.

2. Month: (4 sessions) one individual session of 90 minutes per week together with the clinical psychiatrist and clinical psychologist and cognitive behavioral psychotherapist. Build of therapeutic relationship, psycho-education to the family and reduction of high-expressed emotion, motivational interviewing.

3. Month: (8 sessions) two individual sessions of one hour per week with the clinical psychiatrist and clinical psychologist and cognitive behavioral psychotherapist. Build of therapeutic relationship, psycho-education, motivational interviewing and enhancement of assertiveness to claim their rights.

B. Second phase (160 sessions)

1. Individual psychotherapy (cognitive phase)
CBTp (30 sessions) (once a week 1 hour), CR-T (70 sessions) (once a week, one hour)

2. A pause of 2 months

3. Group psychotherapy (rehabilitation and metacognitive phase)
IPT (50 sessions) (twice a week, each one hour), MCT (10 sessions) (twice a week, each one hour).

C. Third phase (2 months) (8 sessions) (Epilogue)

1. Individual follow-up session weekly of 90 minutes together with the clinical psychiatrist and clinical psychologist and cognitive behavioral psychotherapist and with the person with TRS and the family. Relapse prevention. Recovery as a process.

D. 2 monthly individual sessions are being given as follow-up.

Total number of sessions of RECOVERYTRSGR: 190.

E. Psychometric evaluation regarding cognitive functions, symptoms, social skills, and problem-solving, functional outcome and recovery after the intervention (recovery as an outcome).

F. Psychometric evaluation regarding cognitive functions, symptoms, social skills and problem-solving, functional outcome and recovery in a follow-up after six months (recovery as an outcome).

Fig. 4.1 Recovery-oriented pharmacotherapy and psychotherapy for people with TRS. A Greek model (RECOVERYTRSGR)

4.2 Recovery-Oriented Pharmacotherapy for Treatment-Resistant Schizophrenia a Greek Model (RECOVERYTRSGR)

The first phase of this model is the introductory phase and is carried out by all mental health professionals responsible for the recovery process of the person with TRS (clinical psychiatrist, clinical psychologist, and cognitive-behavioral psychotherapist). This first phase includes 3 months of treatment. Psychological assessment will be performed before intervention regarding intellectual quotient, symptoms, cognitive function, functional outcome, and recovery process.

During the first month, four individual sessions are dedicated to build the therapeutic relationship, conduct motivational interviews, and provide psychoeducation around TRS and the importance of pharmacotherapy. Two 1-h sessions per week are offered, one with a clinical psychiatrist and one with a clinical psychologist and cognitive-behavioral psychotherapist.

During the second month, four weekly sessions of 90 min each with a clinical psychiatrist, clinical psychologist, and cognitive-behavioral psychotherapist are devoted to build therapeutic relationship, motivational interviewing, and psychoeducation by the family of the person with TRS, so that the importance of pharmacotherapy and psychotherapy can be discussed and high expressed emotion of the members can be reduced.

Finally, in the third month, two individual 1-h sessions per week—one with a clinical psychiatrist and a second with a clinical psychologist and cognitive-behavioral psychotherapist, are also devoted to the therapeutic relationship, motivational interviewing on the importance of pharmacotherapy and psychotherapy, and discussion of potential issues with the family of the person with TRS. An introduction to recovery-oriented psychotherapy will be presented. Psychiatrists and psychologists must inform people with TRS of all their rights and how they can exercise them. For example, people with TRS have the right to receive financial support from the government and support through employment. Non-evidence-based pharmacological treatment (polypharmacy) and non-evidence-based psychotherapy should be avoided. If they are victims of misconduct, mental health professionals should help them seek legal help.

All the appropriate medical evaluations should be proceeded, in order to evaluate the possibility of administrating clozapine. If clozapine can be safely administrated, then clozapine therapy can begin. If not, we should alternatively give other antipsychotic agents taking on account the patient's side effects profile. Try not to use more than two agents if possible.

The third phase (epilogue) of RECOVERYTRSGR lasts 2 months. A clinical psychiatrist, clinical psychologist, and psychotherapist work together to provide weekly individual 90-min follow-up sessions for people with TRS and their families to see the impact of the second stage of RECOVERYTRSGR and to relieve the strong emotions of family members. Repeating the process will yield a better assessment.

Finally, *two individual monthly sessions* are offered for follow-up.

In sum, the pharmacotherapy in the context of RECOVERYTRSGR has been described. Pharmacotherapy is the main therapy which is the main condition so that evidence-based psychotherapy can be implemented. A new restart in pharmacotherapy after many unsuccessful sessions of pharmacotherapy in the past is not an easy choice. Clinical experience of psychiatrists is on demand.

4.3 Recovery-Oriented Psychotherapy and Rehabilitation for Treatment-Resistant Schizophrenia. A Greek Model (RECOVERYTRSGR) (Fig. 4.1)

The first phase of this model is the *introductory phase* and is carried out by all mental health professionals responsible for the recovery process of the person with TRS (clinical psychiatrist, clinical psychologist, and cognitive-behavioral psychotherapist). This first phase includes 3 months of treatment. Psychological assessment will be performed before intervention regarding intellectual quotient, symptoms, cognitive function, functional outcome, and recovery process.

During the *first month,* eight weekly individual 1-h sessions are dedicated to build the therapeutic relationship and conduct motivational interviewing and psychoeducation around TRS and the importance of psychotherapy. Two sessions per week are offered, one with a clinical psychiatrist and one with a clinical psychologist and cognitive-behavioral psychotherapist.

During the *second month,* four weekly sessions of 90 min each with a clinical psychiatrist, clinical psychologist, and cognitive-behavioral psychotherapist are devoted to build therapeutic relationships and motivational interviewing and carry out psychoeducation by the family of the person with TRS to be able to discuss the importance of psychotherapy and reduce the emotions that members express presently.

Finally, in the *third month,* eight sessions—two individual 1-h sessions per week—one with a clinical psychiatrist and the second with clinical psychologist and cognitive psychotherapist are also devoted to the therapeutic relationship, motivational interviewing on the importance of pharmacotherapy and of psychotherapy, and discuss potential issues with the family of the person with TRS. An introduction to recovery-oriented psychotherapy will be presented. Psychiatrists and psychologists must inform people with TRS of all their rights and how they can exercise them. For example, people with TRS have the right to receive financial support from the government and support through employment. Non-evidence-based pharmacological treatment (polypharmacy) and non-evidence-based psychotherapy should be avoided. If they are victims of misconduct, mental health professionals should help them seek legal help.

Motivational interviewing is a specific style of communication and collaboration within the therapeutic relationship that focuses on change. The pros and cons of potential changes are discussed. People with specific mental health disorders and TRS have increased motivation to change in the context of acceptance and commitment. Motivational interviewing includes four processes: (1) Engaging: developing a working relationship, (2) Focusing: develop a focus on change during the conversation, (3) Evoking: discussing the motivation for change, (4) Planning: develop a commitment to change and a specific plan of action [21]. Non-adherence to medication treatment and low motivation in psychotherapy can be discussed in motivational interviewing so that people with TRS can find new perspectives on pharmacotherapy and psychotherapy.

Taken together, the first 3 months represent an introductory phase aimed at building the therapeutic relationship and restarting with adequate, evidence-based pharmacotherapy. If suicidal thoughts or plans are ongoing, a cognitive-behavioral intervention specifically related to suicidal ideation should be implemented, as described in the following paragraphs.

The first part of the *second phase* of RECOVERYTRSGR focuses on a long-term combination of evidence-based pharmacotherapy and psychotherapy for people with TRS. It focuses on *individual therapy (cognitive phase)* and a combination of evidence-based individual psychotherapies. The following psychotherapies are recommended: Individual CBTp therapy at a rate of 30 weekly 1-h sessions and CR-T 70 weekly 1-h sessions to better cope with positive and negative symptoms and the resulting distress and reinforce positive beliefs about oneself, which can have a positive impact on managing positive and negative symptoms. Suicide is the first issue that needs to be discussed and resolved in CBTp. We talk about it openly and train people how to deal with it. After 100 sessions, there is a *2-month break* to relax and see the effects of psychotherapy. Psychiatric treatment takes place once a month.

It is very important to start with individual psychotherapy so that people have time to improve and learn to express their difficulties. It is well known that people with TRS are very suspicious and traumatized by frequent and ineffective treatments in the past! This means they first need individual psychotherapy to gain confidence in evidence-based treatments and prepare for the second part, which focuses on group psychotherapy.

Suicidal behavior must be treated with a preventative and therapeutic approach, with openness and transparency, without stereotypes. It is very important to talk about this issue with all people with TRS, regardless of whether they are currently actively suicidal or not. Most of them have faced it in the past, even if they don't have it right now.

A good therapeutic relationship will provide a safe context to talk openly about the issue and respond with empathy and renewed hope. A transparent psychoeducational approach to suicidal behavior by describing thoughts and behaviors and presenting an intervention structure against it and for more hope in life contributes to bringing more transparency, safety, and control to difficult situations. Suicidal therapy is delivered within the context of a cohesive and collaborative therapeutic relationship.

The Five-Step Suicide Assessment and Triage (SAFE-T) (www.sprc.org or www.stopasuicide.org) presents a very effective framework for mental health professionals that include many factors that can be evaluated in full detail and relevance. The following steps are recommended: (1) Identify risk factors. (2) Identify protective factors. (3) Suicide inquiry (suicidal thoughts, plans, behaviors and intent). (4)

Evaluation of risk and choose of the appropriate intervention to cope with the risk, and finally, (5) Documentation (evaluation of risk, intervention, and follow-up).

A suicide prevention contract must be signed between a clinical psychiatrist, clinical psychologist, and cognitive-behavioral psychotherapist and the individual with TRS and suicidal thoughts so that he/she can contact mental health professionals to inform them of the suicidal thoughts, intentions, and plans and to schedule a session with a clinical psychiatrist and clinical psychologist. The above contract reduces impulses toward suicide and social isolation while also sending a central message: People with TRS are not alone and can always find other ways to cope with hallucinations, delusions, depression, and despair.

A person with TRS and suicidal thoughts and behavior feels vulnerable, weak in the face of schizophrenia, isolated and stigmatized, and with luck of control on the disorder. Hallucinations and delusions dictate people's lives and dictate suicidal behavior. A very common example of an acoustic hallucination is a voice telling the person to harm themselves. A person with TRS is often exhausted by schizophrenia, has a poor quality of life, and has no other options in this life but suicide.

CBT is an effective treatment for suicidal tendencies and contributes to reduce suicidal ideation and suicide attempts [22].

CBT educates people with TRS about cognitive interventions and especially about not accepting automatic thoughts related to suicidal ideation as reality. These automatic thoughts are linked to basic cognitive schema, such as vulnerability, weakness, loneliness, abandonment, and control. People with TRS feel very isolated, have delusions and hallucinations, and have no way to cope. CBTp trains them to cope with the distress that arises from these severe symptoms and thus control them. Then, gradually, they feel less vulnerable, weak, and lonely, and they have more control over their TRS and their own lives. Behavioral strategies, such as problem-solving interventions, help them evaluate alternatives to suicidal thoughts, ideas, and plans. CR-T can enhance positive self-beliefs about the ability to implement cognitive and behavioral strategies to cope with suicidal tendencies, and the ability to see new perspectives and meaning in life.

The family of a person with TRS must be informed about the potential danger of suicidal thoughts and attempts if the person has a good relationship with the family and if the family is aware of the person's TRS. Psychoeducation about TRS and suicidal ideation plays an important role.

The second part of the *second phase* of the combination of evidence-based pharmacotherapy and psychotherapy focuses on the combination of *group* evidence-based programs *(rehabilitation and metacognitive phase),* which focus on cognitive distortions that are related with delusions and on rehabilitation regarding cognitive dysfunctions, symptoms, social skills, and problem-solving skills. The second phase of this psychotherapy provides 60 sessions; 50 1-h IPT sessions twice a week followed by ten 1-h MCT sessions twice a week. IPT and MCT will be offered by a clinical psychiatrist, clinical psychologist, and cognitive-behavioral psychotherapist who are trained in these programs. The psychiatric treatment is going on once a month.

The third phase (epilogue) (eight sessions) of RECOVERYTRSGR lasts 2 months. Clinical psychiatrists, clinical psychologists, and psychotherapists work together to provide weekly, 1-h individual follow-up sessions for people with TRS and their families to see the impact of the second stage of RECOVERYTRSGR and reduce the strong emotions of family members. Psycho education in relapse prevention will be provided. Repeating the process will yield a better assessment. The recovery perspective (recovery as a process or subjective recovery) plays an important role in this third phase (epilogue) and is a central theme of the sessions.

Recovery as an outcome or objective recovery means that individuals with TRS should be evaluated with psychometric tests before, after, and in a follow-up of 6 or more months after the end of the therapy.

Recovery as a process or subjective recovery means therapy as a dynamic and ongoing procedure rather than static. Individuals must take responsibility for their own mental health and be protagonists. For example, it may be that people with TRS have improved in many areas, such as anxiety, depression, hallucinations, and cognitive function, but they need more time to cope effectively with delusions.

Finally, *two individual monthly sessions* are offered for follow-up. These sessions are held in collaboration with clinical psychiatrists, clinical psychologists, and people with TRS.

Psychological assessments regarding symptoms, cognitive function, functional outcomes, and recovery will be performed after completion of RECOVERYTRSGR and at 6-month follow-up. Psychiatric treatment takes place once a month. If relapse occurs after 12 months, the combination of pharmacotherapy and evidence-based psychotherapy (RECOVERYTRSGR) above should be repeated.

Total number of sessions of RECOVERYTRSGR: 190

Taken together, the implementation of evidence-based psychotherapy in the context of RECOVERYTRSGR has been described and explained. Suicidality should be treated as a priority before RECOVERYTRSGR is offered. 190 sessions can be offered in total. It is possible to repeat the whole program, if the results are not satisfactory or a relapse has taken place.

4.4 Discussion

TRS presents a distinct category in schizophrenia and is associated with high burden and bad quality of life. Our experience with TRS led us to think about developing a new recovery-oriented model in which all the difficulties are taken into consideration. TRS needs long-term recovery-oriented and evidence-based pharmacotherapy and psychotherapy.

It is very important nowadays to prepare the conditions in order to combine evidence-based treatments [20].

Pharmacotherapy is the main therapy for patients with TRS. A therapeutic relationship that is characterized through empathy, honesty, structure, and goal-oriented behavior presents the context to discuss all the possible previous negative experiences with pharmacotherapy, to make a restart avoiding malpractices of the past, to offer psycho education in TRS, and to enhance the motivation for the appropriate agent, and specifically clozapine.

Psychiatrists should show intensive empathy toward patients with TRS regarding side effects as it can be the main reason of drop-out from the therapeutic process. We must have in mind that rapid discontinuation of clozapine causes a major relapse.

The introduction phase tries to register negative experiences and to contribute to a new restart in a context of evidence-based treatments. The second phase provides effective evidence-based individual and group psychotherapies. The conclusion is a review of all the changes that have been made and improvements related to the quality of life of people with TRS and their families. Finally, two monthly follow-ups aim to separate and assess recovery or subjective recovery. Psychiatric treatment is the main therapy and takes place once a month. Individual and group psychotherapy within the framework of cognitive-behavioral psychotherapy and rehabilitation is an adjunct therapy to pharmacotherapy. A psychological assessment will be given pre-intervention, post-intervention, and at 6-month follow-up (recovery as an outcome).

RECOVERYTRSGR (Fig. 4.1) lasts 190 sessions and teaches people with TRS and their families how to cope with schizophrenia, TRS, and suicidal risk and improves cognitive functions and symptoms, recovery, and functional outcome results. People find new meaning in life after a difficult diagnosis. They learn to consult a stable therapy group for help. This ambulatory setting minimizes the likelihood of hospitalization and increases the likelihood of living in the community in the context of social reintegration focused on recovery.

Mental health professionals should devote themselves to this therapy long term and over many years. This means they must have clinical experience and appropriate training for the long-term treatment of chronic mental health disorders, such as schizophrenia and TRS.

RECOVERYTRSGR (Fig. 4.1) has advantages and disadvantages. Its benefit is that it is a recovery-oriented therapy that includes evidence-based treatments for people with TRS; it protects people from repeated hospitalizations and suicidal behavior; it offers the possibility of repeating the program after 12 months in case of relapse; and it is a good example of the importance of good cooperation between a clinical psychiatrist and a clinical psychologist. Cognitive and metacognitive perspectives are taken into account. Recovery as an outcome and recovery as a process are important parts of this therapy.

The disadvantages are that the program lasts several months, and if collaboration between mental health professionals is not effective, it is difficult to implement. Finally, the cost of treatment is also an issue. In Greece, this program must be paid for by individuals and is not covered by insurance, but it is offered at a low price to make it accessible to these people. The authors implemented the program over the past 10 months in a pilot study on a sample of five people with TRS. It had a positive effect on their lives. Further research studies regarding the efficacy and effectiveness of RECOVERYTRSGR (Fig. 4.1) are in demand.

The comorbidity of TRS and personality disorders presents a very important clinical issue that can be arisen also by the implementation of RECOVERYTRSGR. TRS and borderline personality disorder, antisocial, schizoid, and histrionic personality disorder is one of the most difficult combinations, according to clinical experience. An antisocial personality disorder doesn't accept the rules of society. These people destroy every interpersonal relationship and are dangerous, showing criminal behavior.

A borderline personality disorder shows impulsive, unstable, and auto-destructive behavior. If this impulsive behavior is affected by the positive symptoms, such as hallucinations, this is a very critical situation. A schizoid prefers lonely activities, and this increases the possibility not coming to group therapy. A histrionic personality seeks for attention all the time!

RECOVERYTRSGR begins with a restart of pharmacotherapy and a psychoeducation. Afterward, individual cognitive therapy will be implemented, which gives the chance to restructure the schemas of personality disorders and to change dysfunctional behavioral patterns that are also related to personality disorders. Group cognitive behavior therapy and rehabilitation will be implemented in such a way that patients with TRS feel capable, step by step, of coping with TRS. This enhances the possibility of continuation with group therapy. That means that antisocial, borderline, histrionic, and schizoid personality disorders have more chances in the context of RECOVERYTRSGR to participate on all 190 sessions. The therapeutic relationship that is motivation- and recovery-oriented and activates resources has a positive impact on the above difficult personality disorders.

The following characteristics reduce the possibility of dropping out of RECOVERYTRSGR: the presence of two different mental health experts—a clinical psychologist and a clinical psychiatrist; open communication about any problem that has arisen in the past, such as non-evidence-based pharmacotherapy and psychotherapies; and the side effects of agents. Additionally, the treatment of suicidality as a first priority and the implementation of individual and group psychotherapy contribute to enhance the possibility of remaining with RECOVERYTRSG and carrying on with the therapy.

The application of motivational interviewing throughout the duration of RECOVERYTRSGR can also contribute to the expression of difficulties and the focus on action to solve problems.

In other words, RECOVERYTRSGR takes all the appropriate measures to minimize the possibility of dropping out. On the other hand, dropping out is a part of clinical practice, and we cannot avoid it. Some patients with TRS will not follow our vision! Or they need more time to think about their participation. We accept that, and we carry on with other patients who want to participate in our program.

RECOVERYTRSGR is a very good example of the importance of the close and mutual cooperation of clinical psychiatrists and clinical psychologists. This cooperation is characterized by reciprocity, coherence, and respect for the limits of each specialty. Competition, sabotaging the colleague's work, and sending double messages to the patient with TRS and the family are unethical and can lead to the dissolution of the therapeutic relationship and treatment. These also create relapses in patients, which are also associated with grief after the loss of another therapeutic relationship with mental health experts.

The best and most effective programs suffer from the human factor or from the possibility of unsuccessful cooperation between mental health experts. If they do not cooperate with each other, no treatment program will work as well as RECOVERYTRSGR. So, mental health professionals are responsible for the proper cooperation with each other and for the best possible implementation of RECOVERYTRSGR.

Clinical psychologists and clinical psychiatrists should have completed training in cognitive-behavioral psychotherapy, in CR-T (Beck Institute), in metacognitive training (Prof S. Moritz) and in IPT (Prof. V. Roder), so that they can be trained in our program, the RECOVERYTRSGR, and under these circumstances they can to be able to practice it safely.

Evidence-based psychotherapeutic training of mental health experts increases the possibility of treatment success in RECOVERYTRSGR and the formation of a long-term therapeutic relationship.

RECOVERYTRSGR is a long-term recovery-oriented therapy giving stability, structure, and improvement in specific areas of the life, which are associated with the reintegration into society of patients with TRS. It offers sufficient time to adjust to the new reality and to restart life. Patients and their families construct a stable, long-term therapeutic relationship with mental health experts. A long-term therapeutic relationship enhances the motivation for step-by-step improvement in the daily routine under the guidance of a secure therapeutic relationship.

RECOVERYTRSGR highlights the advantages of the synthesis of evidence-based interventions for TRS with the probability of a repetition of the therapy in case of a relapse. It is an integrated therapeutic program centered on different levels, such as cognitive dysfunctions, symptoms, and functional outcomes. An integrated program is able to treat, step-by-step, all the resistant dysfunctions, symptoms, and suicidality.

RECOVERYTRSGR gives TRS patients and their families an understanding of the difficulties of TRS, the consequences of it all these years, why patients feel so desperate to manage TRS, what measures should be taken by pharmacotherapy in order to avoid polypharmacy and side effects and which evidence-based psychotherapies should be chosen and why. Treatment-resistant cognitive dysfunctions present a main issue. Therefore, patients with TRS need more time to learn, to restructure their beliefs regarding their lives, and to adapt to a new reality!

RECOVERYTRSGR gives patients with TRS and their families hope for a new restart in life. Chronic mental health disorders, such as TRS, are confronted with deep grief throughout their lives. RECOVERYTRSGR contributes to the transformation of grief, hopelessness, weakness and loneliness to hope, action for life, strength, and cohesion with other people, such as mental health experts and family members.

The therapeutic relationship in the context of RECOVERYTRSGR is motivation-, disclosure-, and recovery-oriented. Every session contributes to the enhancement of the possibility of change. The advantages and disadvantages for every potential of change and progress will be discussed. Problems and negative emotions will be expressed without stereotypes so that patients with TRS and their families can reduce their vulnerability. Grief displays a very important issue.

The long-term grief regarding the relapses, the long-term hospitalizations, and the non-adherence to pharmacotherapy and what this means in the past, in the present, and in the future will be expressed and analyzed. A difficult situation, such as TRS, presents a challenge to reevaluate this chronic mental health disorder, to change the whole life and the interpersonal relationships, to adapt to a new reality with realistic expectations, and finally, to be the protagonist of the own difficult situation. That means that patients with TRS will take the responsibility to change things step by step in life with hope, activation of resources, and flexibility.

The socioeconomic situation in Greece is not sustainable for its citizens. Greece was confronted with a deep economic crisis from 2007 until today, which affected the whole country and especially the health system. The Greek health system doesn't cover the cost of psychotherapeutic sessions.

Patients with TRS and other mental health disorders can participate in psychotherapy in the public mental health sectors without financial burden or pay for the psychotherapeutic sessions themselves in the private mental health sector. Patients with TRS need another alternative in order to cover the cost of psychotherapeutic sessions. RECOVERYTRSGR displays an alternative for these people and is adapted to the needs of patients with TRS in Greece.

RECOVERYTRSGR offers psychotherapeutic sessions at very low prices and is adapted to the difficult socioeconomic situation of Greece and of TRS. Patients with TRS are confronted very early with the disorder and they don't have the chance to achieve important life goals. The majority of them are very poor in Greece and take a small amount of social and financial support that doesn't cover the main costs of their lives.

RECOVERYTRSGR will try to fill a hole in Greece and in other countries with respect to the implementation of evidence-based interventions by patients with TRS and their families. Greek scientists follow the international evidence-based therapeutic guidelines regarding pharmacotherapy for patients with TRS. The absence of an integrated therapeutic model for these people in Greece and also in other countries, which combines recovery-oriented pharmacotherapy and psychotherapy, presents a reality. Hence, we trust that our program will fill this hole within the scientific community.

Our long-term experiences with TRS have highlighted the problems with this disorder all these years in Greece. Hence, we have decided to develop this recovery-oriented program taking into account all the problems of TRS: treatment resistance, relapses, hospitalizations, suicidal crises, and non-adherence to the treatments, ECT as a choice and difficulties with that, and huge problems in the interfamilial relationships. A long-term, goal-oriented, and recovery-oriented integrative program will be the solution to the above-mentioned problems.

It gives enough space and time to talk about the negative experiences in the past, to evaluate the dysfunctional choices in pharmacotherapy in the past, to talk openly about clozapine and other agents, to make a restart in pharmacotherapy, to explain the advantages of every cognitive-behavioral psychotherapy and rehabilitation in RECOVERYTRSGR, and to implement them step by step.

The family plays an important role in the therapy. 190 sessions with the possibility of repetition in case of a relapse present a very motivation-oriented context to prepare the situation for change and transformation in order to achieve a better reintegration into society. A long-term therapeutic relationship will be developed in order to treat the problems of the past, find solutions in the present, and to be a protective umbrella for future crises and relapses.

The maintenance of the therapeutic relationship with the patients with TRS and their families even after the completion of RECOVERYTRSGR is a very important fact. These patients need time to learn and put them into practice. The possibility of repeating the program after a relapse also meets the basic needs of TRS.

Greece has been going through a socioeconomic from 2008 until today. Greece has many structural problems and does not invest enough funds in the field of health. Our program can be a possibility for evidence-based intervention in combination with the evaluation of its effectiveness and efficacy.

Taken together, RECOVERYTRSGR presents an overview of evidence-based treatments in TRS. The introduction phase tries to register negative experiences. The second phase provides effective evidence-based individual and group psychotherapies. The conclusion is a review of all the changes that have been made. Finally, two monthly follow-ups aim to separate and assess recovery, or subjective recovery. It lasts for 190 sessions. It has advantages and disadvantages. Recovery as an outcome and recovery as a process are important parts of this therapy. Finally, RECOVERYTRSGR contributes to the transformation of grief, hopelessness, weakness, and loneliness into hope, action for life, strength, and cohesion with others.

4.5 Conclusions

RECOVERYTRSGR presents a new proposal for the long-term treatment of TRS. This has advantages and disadvantages. Future studies on the effectiveness and efficacy of this model are required.

Revision Questions

1. Describe the new recovery-oriented pharmacotherapy (RECOVERYTRSGR) for TRS
2. Describe the new recovery-oriented psychotherapy (RECOVERYTRSGR) for TRS
3. Which is the new element in this new model (RECOVERYTRSGR)?
4. What are its advantages and disadvantages?

Competing Interests The authors have no conflicts of interest to declare that are relevant to the content of this chapter.

The authors organize an annual training on the new recovery-oriented therapy for treatment-resistant schizophrenia (RECOVERYTRSGR) for clinical psychologists, clinical psychiatrists, and cognitive behavioral psychotherapists. For more information, please visit https://www.linkedin.com/in/stavroula-rakitzi-0b512b45/, http://orcid.org/0000-0002-5231-6619 (Stavroula Rakitzi), https://gr.linkedin.com/in/polyxeni-georgila-940b521a7, http://orcid.org/0000-0003-3137-506x (Polyxeni Georgila) or email srakitzi@gmail.com.

References

1. Yang AC, Tsai SJ. New targets for schizophrenia treatment beyond the dopamine hypothesis. Int J Mol Sci. 2017;18:1689. https://doi.org/10.3390/ijms18081689.
2. Zubin J, Spring BJ. Vulnerability—a new view of schizophrenia. J Abnorm Psychol. 1977;86:103–26.
3. Green MF, Nuechterlein KH. Should schizophrenia be treated as a neurocognitive disorder? Schizophr Bull. 1999;25(2):309–18.
4. Schmidt SJ, Mueller DR, Roder V. Social cognition as a mediator between neurocognition and functional outcome in schizophrenia: empirical review and new results by structural equation modelling. Schizophr Bull. 2011;37(2):41–54.
5. Brenner HD, Hodel B, Roder V, Corrigan P. Treatment of cognitive dysfunctions and behavioral deficits in schizophrenia: integrated psychological therapy. Schizophr Bull. 1992;18:21–6.
6. Nuecterlein KH, Green MF. MATRICS consensus cognitive battery. Los Angeles: MATRICS Assessment Inc.; 2006.
7. Kay SR, Fiszbein A, Opler LA. The positive and negative syndrome scale (PANSS) for schizophrenia. Schizopr Bull. 1987;13(2):261–76.
8. Lykouras L, Botsis A, Oulis P. The PANSS scale. Athens: Scientific Publications; 2005.
9. World Health Organization. International classification of functioning, disability and health (ICF). Geneva: World Health Organization; 2001.
10. Koumpouros Y, Papageorgiou E, Sakellari E, et al. Adaptation and psychometric properties evaluation of the Greek version of WHODAS 2.0. Pilot application in Greek elderly population. Health Serv Outcomes Res Methodol. 2018;18(1):63–74. https://doi.org/10.1007/s10742-017-0176-x.
11. Hancock N, Scanlan JN, Bundy AC, Honey A. Recovery Assessment Scale-Domains & Stages (RAS-DS) manual-version 3. Sydney: University of Sydney; 2019.
12. Hancock N, the University of Sydney, Rakitzi S. Katoudi S. Recovery Assessment Scale-Domains & Stages (RAS-DS). The Greek version; 2023.
13. Aster M, Neubauer M, Horn R. Wechsler-Intelligenztest für Erwachsene WIE. Frankfurt: Harcourt Test Services; 2006.
14. Beck AT, Rector NA, Stolar N, Grant P. Schizophrenia. Cognitive theory, research and therapy. New York: The Guilford Press; 2009.
15. Beck AT, Grant P, Inverso E, Brinen AP, Perivoliotis D. Recovery oriented cognitive therapy for serious mental health conditions. New York: The Guilford Press; 2021.
16. Roder V, Mueller DR, Schmidt SJ. Effectiveness of Integrated Psychological Therapy (IPT) for schizophrenia patients. Schizophr Bull. 2011;37(Suppl. 2):71–9. https://doi.org/10.1093/schbul/sbr072.
17. Mueller DH, Schmidt SJ, Roder V. Integrated psychological therapy. Effectiveness in schizophrenia inpatient settings related to patients age. Am J Geriatr Psychiatry. 2013;21(3):231–41. https://doi.org/10.1016/j.jagp.2012.12.011.
18. Moritz S, Menon M, Balzan R, Woodward TS. Metacognitive training for psychosis (MCT): past, present and future. Eur Archiv Psychiatry Clin Neurosci. 2022;273:811. https://doi.org/10.1007/s00406-022-01394-9.
19. Penney D, Sauvé G, Mendelson D, Thibaudeau E, Moritz S, Lepage M. Immediate and sustained outcomes and moderators associated with metacognitive training for psychosis. A systematic review and meta-analysis. JAMA Psychiatry. 2022;79:417. https://doi.org/10.1001/jamapsychiatry.2022.0277.
20. Rakitzi S. Clinical psychology and cognitive behavioral psychotherapy. Recovery in mental health. Cham, Switzerland: Springer; 2023.
21. Miller WR, Rollnick S. Application of motivational interviewing. Motivational interviewing: helping people change. New York: Guilford Press; 2013.
22. Wu H, Lu L, Qian Y, Jin XH, Yu HR, Du L, Fu XL, ZhuB CHL. The significance of cognitive-behavioral therapy on suicide. An umbrella review. J Affect Disord. 2022;317:142–8. https://doi.org/10.1016/j.jad.2022.08.067.

Epilogue 5

TRS is one of the most challenging chronic mental health disorders. Today, we cannot blame the fact that evidence-based pharmacotherapy, psychotherapy, and rehabilitation are not available to these people. Research is also continuing and should yield positive results in a few years in terms of pharmacotherapy and psychotherapy.

TRS presents a distinct category of schizophrenia. Our experience with TRS led us to think about developing a new, recovery-oriented model. TRS needs long-term recovery-oriented and evidence-based pharmacotherapy and psychotherapy.

TRS is a challenge for all of us. We have to be devoted to these individuals in the long term and show deep empathy for them. They have been traumatized in the past by many non-evidence-based treatments and have lost faith in mental health experts.

Empirical data regarding the efficacy of pharmacotherapy in TRS shows us the way. Clozapine is the treatment of first choice if it can be administered without negative medical consequences. The appropriate pharmacotherapy for TRS presents the right context, and after 3 months, experts can continue with recovery-oriented psychotherapy and rehabilitation. This goal-oriented and structured way will decrease the possibility of relapse and suicidal risk in the future.

Research regarding new agents for schizophrenia and TRS is in process, and we expect new medications and possibly genetic therapies in the future. *Genetic therapies will eliminate the root of this disorder. On the other hand, it is very difficult to find an exact genetic therapy that will root out the treatment-resistant positive and negative symptoms as well as the treatment-resistant cognitive dysfunction.*

Until this day comes, we have to be patient and carry on with the available long-term evidence-based interventions for patients with TRS. RECOVERYTRSGR displays an opportunity in that direction and can also support patients with TRS in case of the existence of genetic therapies.

Long-term treatment that focuses on recovery will help them regain confidence in their treatment. Long-term outpatient treatment focused on recovery will help them find new meaning in life, avoid unnecessary hospitalizations, claim all rights

S. Rakitzi, P. Georgila, *Treatment-Resistant Schizophrenia*,
https://doi.org/10.1007/978-3-031-64623-2_5

to better reintegrate into society, and become protagonists in their own lives in the context of recovery.

Polypharmacy, side effects due to polypharmacy, and the execution of non-evidence-based treatments display traumatic experiences for patients with TRS. They need much more time to make a new restart in the context of evidence-based therapy. As mental health experts, we are obliged to have the appropriate training and clinical experience as clinical psychologists, clinical psychiatrists, and cognitive behavioral psychotherapists with patients with TRS and with evidence-based treatments.

Why should polypharmacy be chosen? What are the criteria? Are the criteria scientific and evidence-based? Why should non-evidence-based psychotherapy for TRS be chosen? What are the criteria? Are the criteria scientific and evidence-based? All the above questions ought to be addressed to patients with TRS and their families, who are victims of the above strategies. Could a very bad relapse due to polypharmacy and non-evidence-based psychotherapies lead to a big trauma and post-traumatic stress disorder? Yes, of course. May a distressing relapse lead to suicide? Yes, unfortunately!

One of the biggest traumas of patients with TRS and their families is one of the most unethical behaviors of mental health experts: the sexual abuse of individuals with TRS by mental health experts. Patients build a therapeutic relationship with experts, which is a bridge to learning new things and reintegrating into society. If mental health experts abuse this relationship in order to have a sexual relationship with the patients, then this is an entryway to suicidality. This trauma needs many years to be cured and to be replaced by a secure and stable life with reasonable objective goals.

TRS patients, who are stood up to with polypharmacy, non-evidence-based interventions, and the trauma of sexual abuse from mental health experts, present a distinct category of individuals with TRS, which we treated all these years. It is continuously exceptionally troublesome as well as outstanding for us to offer evidence-based interventions to these people. They are real fighters and merit our admiration and commitment. They need to bargain with numerous traumas synchronically and find a balance within the setting of TRS.

Our book could be a journey to evidence-based treatments for patients with TRS and their families. It is composed in a way that is reasonable to non-experts. Hence, we want to help these people know the truth about TRS, the complications that are related to it, the evidence-based interventions that are accessible, how to avoid malpractice by mental health experts and what are their human rights regarding the access to recovery-oriented treatments.

Governments in all over the world ought to fund psychotherapy for mental health disorders through insurances. Recovery-oriented treatments should be covered. Clinics, ambulant settings and private practice must offer only evidence-based treatments to individuals with mental health disorders, and especially TRS.

The Greek insurance system doesn't cover psychotherapy, and there is no intention toward such an objective, which is exceptionally dangerous and disappointing. Greek psychiatric departments in clinics, ambulant settings in the public and private sectors, and private practices in Greece should be evaluated through Greek governments and Greek scientific associations to determine whether they offer evidence-based treatments and how effective and efficacious their implementation of these therapies is. RECOVERYTRSGR can fill this gap in Greece and in other countries. GREECE does not offer adequate financial support for research in mental health.

RECOVERYTRSGR, a new ambulant program focused on recovery, is leading the way. It consists of three phases and gradually prepares the scene for a new restart of pharmacotherapy and psychotherapy. Cognitive, metacognitive, and recovery perspectives play an important role in the structure of the therapy.

The introduction phase tries to register negative experiences and contribute to a new restart in the context of evidence-based treatments. The second phase provides effective evidence-based individual and group psychotherapies. The conclusion is a review of all the changes that have been made. Finally, 2 month follow-ups aim to separate and assess recovery, or subjective recovery. Psychiatric treatment is the main therapy and takes place once a month. Individual and group psychotherapy within the framework of cognitive behavioral psychotherapy and rehabilitation is an adjunct therapy to pharmacotherapy. A psychological assessment will be given pre-intervention, post-intervention, and at 6-month follow-up (recovery as an outcome).

RECOVERYTRSGR lasts 190 sessions and teaches people with TRS and their families how to cope with schizophrenia, TRS, and suicidal risk, improving cognitive functions and symptoms, recovery, and functional outcome results. This ambulatory setting minimizes the likelihood of hospitalization and increases the likelihood of living in the community in the context of social reintegration focused on recovery.

We hope that RECOVERYTRSGR will inspire us and other colleagues to implement it more systematically and evaluate its effectiveness and efficacy.

RECOVERYTRSGR gives the opportunity to build step by step a secure and stable therapeutic relationship that gives opportunities for discussing openly about problems with TRS, with past non-evidence-based treatments, with limits in the context of the therapeutic relationship, and to give patients with TRS enough time and space to probe the changes and to adapt them step by step on their daily routine. The therapeutic relationship in the context of RECOVERYTRSGR is motivation-oriented, goal-oriented with certain limits, and activates the appropriate resources by patients with TRS in order to carry on with the recovery as a process. This therapeutic relationship contributes to the awareness of the problem via *systematic psychoeducation and to the change of the main problems, such as symptoms, cognitive dysfunctions, and dysfunctional thoughts and schemas that have a negative impact on quality of life and functional outcomes. Finally, this relationship transforms the grief regarding TRS into action for life.*

People with TRS and their families need more time to learn, cope with challenges, and find their own rhythm in life within the context of evidence-based treatments.

Grief presents a huge problem. Patients with TRS and their families spend many years grieving the existence of the disorder. The five stages of grief, shock, denial, anger, depression, and acceptance-reboot show a better way to manage this burden and its consequences. Patients manifest to express their grief with psychotic symptoms and family members with chronic depression. Our first contact with them always has almost the same characteristics: relapses, hospitalizations that did not go well, anger, and despair. We become listeners to this pain and grief. We must, before starting any intervention, give space and time for this burden to be expressed.

Grief management has advantages and disadvantages. Disadvantages focus on the fact that, in short term, depression may occur and there may be poor adherence to treatment. The advantages of long-term are greater. This emotional burden has been given a chance to express itself and not continually lead to relapse. The process of acceptance and restart helps in long term to better manage the disorder and to take individual responsibility for mental health improvement.

It is possible to fight against TRS and learn to cope without becoming disorganized, without strong suicidal risk, and without stigma. The new meaning of life is to become a good master of your own problems!

Grief management also helps better manage the stigma of the mental health disorders. The burden surrounding the mental disorder is expressed and, at the same time, given the opportunity to be placed in the person's memory and soul in a context that will not disrupt the person's daily life. Thus, the person accepts himself/herself and his disorder better, and does not feel ashamed or hopeless, does not isolate himself/herself, and looks for ways to live with this disorder. Therefore, the stigma against the disorder is reduced. RECOVERYTRSGR is an action for life and focuses on step-by-step improvement on many levels, such as cognitive, emotional, and behavioral level, and this procedure contributes to a better coping with the disorder and its grief as well as with the stigma regarding TRS.

RECOVERYTRSGR can also help patients with TRS and severe personality disorders. If patients learn to cope with TRS and to restructure schemas that are associated with the psychopathology, this would also have a positive impact on their personality disorder. CBTp and CR-T reduces the burden of dysfunctional schemas, which are also associated with personality disorders. Cognitive restructuring, behavior modification, and social skills that are included in RECOVERYTRSGR are also effective for the treatment of personality disorders. Additionally, the long-term implementation of our therapy in 190 sessions gives us enough space and time to focus indirectly on schemas and behaviors that are associated with personality disorders. On the other hand, RECOVERYTRSGR has as a first priority the treatment of TRS but can intervene indirectly also on the level of personality disorders. It is also known and clear from the clinical practice that when TRS is being treated well, this has a positive impact on the level of dysfunctions in personality.

When patients with TRS are confronted with traumas, such as physical, sexual, and psychological abuse, it is recommended to work very carefully with traumas, implementing cognitive restructuring of thoughts and beliefs and not exposure to trauma. Exposure can lead to a relapse, specifically to a psychotic episode with a suicidal crisis and hospitalization.

A balance between benefits and costs should always be our main orientation when choosing the best possible interventions for TRS in cases of trauma. The worse scenario, according to our clinical practice, is the abuse of patients with TRS by parents or family members, and by mental health experts.

A mental health expert, whom the patient with TRS trusted, built a therapeutic relationship with him and tried through it to change things and improve his quality of life, abused his trust and abused him/her. It is the worst form of abuse of power. Scientific companies are called upon to enable patients to report incidents of violence and to support them in addressing the prosecutorial and judicial authorities. The trauma of abuse always remains deeply rooted within the psychotic symptoms. It takes years to make it manageable, as well as a new reboot with it.

Let's respect the chronicity of TRS and its burden. Let's respect the fact that it is the most difficult chronic mental disorder with a high possibility of suicide. Let us respect the fact that some of our fellow citizens develop, during their lifetime, a chronic mental disorder with a high rate of disability and a high risk of suicide.

The quality of our democracy is assessed by how well it can extend a safety net to our vulnerable fellow citizens, how well it shows them the way of protection from possible abuse of power, and the opportunities it gives them to rehabilitate and reintegrate into society.

The European Union is asked to evaluate all its members who received funds to strengthen mental health services. The questions that arise are the following: How much money did each country get, and where was it channeled? Are evidence-based interventions implemented, and is their effectiveness evaluated? Are there safeguards against abuse of power, and how are they implemented?

The European Union must be the matrix of democracy, which will protect itself and without the citizen having to make reports about whether our vulnerable fellow citizens, such as patients with TRS, are protected by the member states. Specifically in Greece, are evidence-based interventions being implemented in mental health services (public and private sector), is polypharmacy avoided in patients with TRS, under which conditions is ECT applied by patients with TRS?

RECOVERYTRSGR protects patients with TRS from multiple traumas, such as polypharmacy, *ECT,* non-evidence-based psychotherapy in the past and abusive behaviors of mental health experts. Patients know which interventions are going to be offered, in what order, and which therapeutic objectives are planned to be accomplished with every intervention. Two mental health experts are available during the whole process and are obliged to work professionally. Abusive behaviors have no put in our recovery program.

RECOVERYTRSGR has many advantages. Specific evidence-based psychiatric and psychotherapeutic treatments are being offered in one program. Long-term implementation gives the mental health experts a huge chance to improve the resistant cognitive dysfunctions, the positive and negative symptoms, the psychopathology and the functional outcome, and to see the advance of these improvements over the time.

A therapeutic relationship with these people is built through our program, step-by-step, in a secure environment, in which patients know precisely what they are doing and why. They have the right to express their difficulties with the treatment, to declare more help from the experts, and to set their claim limits, in case something is not right for them. Mental health experts are there to teach patients with TRS making a wonderful scientific journey.

In other words, RECOVERYTRSGR upgrades democratic conditions and dismisses each form of abuse by mental health experts to patients with TRS and their families.

Treatment discontinuation is a huge problem in TRS. RECOVERYTRSGR has the following characteristics, which reduce the possibility of treatment interruption: the cohesive collaboration of two different mental health experts-a clinical psychologist and a clinical psychiatrist; an honest communication about any problem, such as non-evidence-based pharmacotherapy and psychotherapies; and the side effects of agents. Additionally, the treatment of suicidality as a first priority and the implementation of individual and group psychotherapy enhance the motivation for remaining at RECOVERYTRSGR. The application of motivational interviewing throughout the duration of RECOVERYTRSGR also enhances the motivation for the therapy.

On the other hand, dropping out is a part of clinical practice, and we cannot avoid it. Some patients with TRS will not follow our vision! Or they need more time to think about their participation.

RECOVERYTRSGR could be described as a person, who enters a chaotic room, in which everything is in disarray, trampled all over the place, torn, and dirty. The person will learn to throw away the worn and useless items, enlist the help of a cleaning crew to clean the space, and then place the useful items inside. Finally, the person will configure the room appropriately so that he/she can stay or go whenever he/she wants and spend his/her time. This room will not cause anxiety, anger, disgust, or psychotic symptoms. It will be a place of calm and safety, in which things will be put in working order and in the appropriate drawers. It will be place that proves that action in life leads to order, calmness, and acceptance of difficult situations.

This room offers peace and security. These conditions will help in a better and cooler management of everyday life, in the better assertion of his rights, as well as in better protection from abuse and professional unethical behavior.

Things are put in order, and this order leads to the improvement of TRS with limits, rules and possibilities for development through the activation of resources. The above conditions are the best conditions for dealing with any incidents of patient abuse.

Patients with TRS are empowered through treatment and know how to distinguish between evidence-based interventions and non-evidence-based treatments. RECOVERYTRSGR shows a structured and transparent psychotherapeutic path to improve functional outcomes and quality of life. Structure and transparency empowers problem-solving as well as resistance to any form of abuse by mental health professionals.

RECOVERYTRSGR displays the importance of the close and mutual cooperation of clinical psychiatrists and clinical psychologists, which is characterized by reciprocity, coherence, and respect. Competition, sabotaging the colleague's work, and sending double messages to the patient with TRS and the family are unethical and can lead to the dissolution of the therapeutic relationship and treatment. Competition and sabotage have no place in the face of the psychological and emotional burden from TRS. The value and dignity of human life are far more important than the competition and selfishness among mental health experts.

The basic prerequisite for the application of the RECOVERYTRSGR by clinical psychologists and clinical psychiatrists is a completed training in cognitive behavioral psychotherapy, in CR-T (Beck Institute), in metacognitive training (Prof S. Moritz), and in IPT (Prof. V. Roder), so that they can be trained afterward by us in our program-the RECOVERYTRSGR. Evidence-based psychotherapeutic training of mental health experts increases the possibility of treatment success in RECOVERYTRSGR.

Patients with TRS and their families who took part in the pilot group of RECOVERYTRSGR have communicated the following impressions:

A. 190 sessions! So many sessions? I was anxious at the beginning because 190 sessions are a long period. I had negative experiences with mental health experts in the past, and so I was exceptionally suspicious. At the conclusion of the treatment, I had the feeling that I could control my serious mental health disorder. It was worth it.
B. I have improved my concentration and memory, and I can better understand social interactions. I have more motivation to appreciate my life and to realize my future goals.
C. I have taken part in numerous psychotherapies *that* last few years. RECOVERYTRSGR has helped me to understand the negative effects of TRS in my life, how psychotherapy works, and that I am also responsible for my mental health each day. I hope that the Greek insurance system will cover the cost of this psychotherapy in the future.
D. The combination of individual and group therapy is fascinating. My family has caught on to me better and shows more empathy for me. The verbal and psychological abuse toward me has been hindered. Dr. Georgila and Dr. Rakitzi are my new family members.
E. I have learned that there are numerous accessible treatments for TRS. I fight in 190 sessions to improve my mental health. It is like a marathon. Interesting *journey*. I have made new friends, who have the same issue as me. Transparency, cohesion, and goal-oriented behavior helped me to build a new relationship with TRS and with my family.
F. I feel more grounded as the mother of a son with TRS to manage this serious mental health disorder. We fight together every day with dignity, love, and cohesion.
G. *A patient with TRS who dropped out due an additional diagnosis of cancer was very happy about his participation on TRS. 120 sessions helped me to understand the disorder and its consequences better and to cope better with them. The cancer diagnosis has changed all the daily routine and that's the reason I didn't do all the sessions of this therapy. RECOVERYTRSGR helped me to cope with the cancer better.*

H. *My Grief was an immense darkness for me. Now I know the truth about TRS, its consequences, and I try every day with my daughter to achieve new goals.*
I. *TRS is the cancer of mental health. The difference is that it lasts a lifetime. My son had a very difficult time with hospitalizations, constant suicidality and no one could ever explain the difficulties of resistant schizophrenia and why it IS RESISTANT. RECOVERYTRSGR showed me a way and taught us to transform our despair and grief into action for life and continuous improvement of the conditions of our life improvement.*
J. *190 sessions! How can be possible that my son will participate? My son dropped out from most of the treatments and didn't take his pharmacotherapy. He believed that psychotherapy is a waste of time! A friend of mine proposed us to contact Dr. Georgila and Dr. Rakitzi. My son made some individual sessions by both of them, in order to enhance his motivation.*

   He decided then to try to take part on RECOVERYTRSGR. As he says, this therapy is something different because we discuss everything, and we try to solve all together problems. So, I feel very happy about the fact that my son found a place to feel safe and to express the negative thoughts.

A patient who participated in RECOVERYTRSGR has decided to write a letter to our recovery-oriented therapy:

Dear RECOVERYTRSGR,

I wanted to die by suicide for many years. I have gone to numerous mental health experts who have prescribed many medications. I slept all day, and the rest of the day I smoked and consumed a lot of junk food. I was very desperate with respect to my life and daily routine. I attempted to find a job, without success.

A friend of mine who suffers from TRS has referred me to Dr. Georgila and Dr. Rakitzi. I met them in three sessions to arrange to clarify how RECOVERYTRSGR can offer assistance to me. I decided to start with this therapy.

I have learned what the issues of TRS are, why I took so numerous medications from past psychiatrists, why clozapine helped me, and how the absence of side effects of pharmacotherapy progressed my quality of life.

Psychotherapy had shown me techniques to manage anxiety, depression, luck of motivation, with delusions and hallucinations. I have to be watch myself each day, like with pharmacotherapy. I am very happy when I accomplish little objectives. I made follow-up sessions with Dr. Georgila and Dr. Rakitzi when I feel overpowered.

I have moved forward my relationship with my family, and especially with my brother. We spend a parcel of time all together without terrible communication and verbal abuse.

I am exceptionally pleased with myself that I battle each day against TRS. I know the truth now and the results of it in my life. There's always a way to manage the negative consequences of a mental health disorder, and that's what I have learned with RECOVERYTRSGR.

The mother of the patient who participated on RECOVERYTRSGR has chosen, moreover, to type in a letter to our recovery-oriented therapy:

Dear RECOVERYTRSGR,

Despair, weakness, entrapment, a mental health death—these words portray my feelings as psychiatrists have announced me the diagnosis of schizophrenia by my son. I was in a long-term grief and severe depression for many years.

My son took a lot of medications and couldn't stay alone at home. He was depressed, slept a lot of hours, wanted to die by suicide, smoked all day and was exceptionally disconnected. I have misplaced my trust that mental health experts can help us.

A friend of my son has proposed that we visit Dr. Georgila and Dr. Rakitzi. I didn't need to meet new mental health experts! My son wanted it, and therefore we decided as a family to make a new beginning with the therapy.

190 sessions! Amazing! I communicate better with my son. We spend more time together, helping him to come to his objectives. My depression has decreased. My son learned that he suffers from a subcategory of schizophrenia, the TRS. He learned to manage with many symptoms and improved his cognitive functions.

He found a new meaning in his life since he was taught a straightforward, structured, and scientific therapy. It is clear for us that polypharmacy isn't essential, that side effects bring more problems, and that we have the right to fight against malpractice.

TRS can be coped with like other health and mental health problems. Participation in a long-term therapeutic program presents the key to enhancement. I am very proud of my son and of my family that we have achieved cohesion, harmony, and a restart in our lives!

A patient who participated in RECOVERYTRSGR has also chosen to compose a letter to our recovery-oriented therapy:

I'm going back 10 years ago. I was diagnosed with schizophrenia and was hospitalized three times in a psychiatric clinic. Since then, I have been treated by a psychiatrist every 15 days. He was prescribed me three anti-psychotic agents, an anti-depressant agent, and an anxiolytic agent. I didn't feel very well and I had suicidal thoughts all the time. He referred me to a psychoanalyst.

I did psychoanalysis for 4 years, two times a week, and my psychotherapy was paid for by my mother. I used to go and talk to myself. At one point, I told the psychoanalyst that the therapy was not helping me. My mother couldn't bear to pay for psychotherapy anymore. He was watching me get worse. My parents searched and found information about RECOVERYTRSGR. So I decided to go and make a new psychotherapy start.

RECOVERYTRSGR has rules, limits and makes sense. I have understood from the first time why polypharmacy didn't help, what TRS is, why psychoeducation is important, why the collaboration with the family is important, and why individual and group cognitive behavioral psychotherapy and rehabilitation is important for TRS.

In other words, I know what my problem is, how it can be expressed, and what I can do to cope with it. This has given me hope and contributed to cope better with my depression.

The parents of a young girl with schizophrenia who participated in RECOVERYTRSGR wrote the following letter:

Our daughter's adolescence was very difficult. She had a lot of anxiety and phobias; she couldn't concentrate on his lessons, and he was causing trouble at school. She was telling us that the devil would come out of the television. We thought these were expressions in the context of puberty. At 20, she made two suicide attempts and was hospitalized two times until she was 22. The diagnosis of schizophrenia scared us a lot. She came out of the hospitals with many drugs and many side effects. At the same time, the psychiatrists changed the agents every week. So we looked for a mental health service in the private sector for her to do psychotherapy. We heard about RECOVERYTRSGR. The explanation of the problems, the reduction of the agents, and the structured framework of psychotherapy helped us all to make a restart. We understood what TRS means.

The psychoeducation as well as the collaborative nature of RECOVERYTRSGR gave us the chance to express our grief, which was transformed into hope and resilience with Dr. Rakitzi and Dr. Georgila. Our daughter has participated in all the sessions of RECOVERYTRSGR and after that, she is more motivated to do things. She is going to carry on with new life goals. The most important thing is that suicidal moments are no longer a daily issue for us. She managed to cope with them very well.

A mother of a patient with TRS has composed the following letter to RECOVERYTRSGR:

Dear RECOVERYTRSGR

I am the mother of a person with TRS. I have visited all the hospitals in Athens, both public and private. My daughter was fine for 2 months, then she didn't want to follow the pharmacotherapy and didn't keep up with the psychiatrists. I had to get a court order for her to be hospitalized for suicidality. I felt the despair of the doctors and psychologists regarding the therapy of my daughter. A psychiatrist suggested ECT. We did that too. My daughter was worsening after ECT. She became disorganized, she couldn't concentrate on anyone or anything, and she couldn't remember anything.

Then I too began to believe that her death would be redemption. He was asking me to be euthanized. I refuse it. I heard about RECOVERYTRSGR and made a contact with Dr. Georgila and Dr. Rakitzi.

The treatment started all over again. We went back to clozapine which was effective. The psychotherapy started step by step, and I saw small changes during the time. Initially, I accompanied my daughter to the sessions because she was not motivated. After 2 months, she went alone.

She described the treatment as a game of exercises. She felt that she was slowly able to manage the suicidal thoughts and auditory hallucinations; she learned to do things that pleased her and improved her mood, and distracted her from the thoughts and hallucinations. She also learned from others in the group. She developed social relations with some of the members of the groups. Life had gained meaning. She tried to improve herself every day.

So her despair went away, and she found a way to become a key partner of mental health experts. She felt her individual responsibility in her treatment.

I personally went through chronic grief for over 10 years. I was on antidepressants and psychotherapy, which helped. These were not enough. I will never forget my daughter's wish for euthanasia, which is not allowed in Greece, the multiple hospitalizations in various psychiatric hospitals, the hopelessness of the doctors and psychologists, but also the change of perspective that was offered through the RECOVERYTRSGR. There is always a way to build an appropriate context to treat TRS. My motivation for life has increased, and I wish that I remain healthy to support my daughter the next years.

A patient who participated in RECOVERYTRSGR but dropped out has chosen to compose a letter to our recovery-oriented therapy:

Dear RECOVERYTRSGR,

All I remember are the hospitalizations. At one point, I was told that I suffer from a severe form of schizophrenia. They didn't explain which one. They gave me a lot of agents. I had side effects. All I remember is that I kept cutting them off and being hospitalized. My parents heard about the RECOVERYTRSGR.

I didn't want to participate. In the end, I said to try because they threatened me with hospitalization. The treatment was very difficult, but I managed. I liked it because it helped my memory and my negative thoughts and it improved my mood.

The parents of the above patient have also composed a letter to RECOVERYTRSGR.

Dear RECOVERYTRSGR,

Our despair and grief had taken over us since our son was 18, when he had his first psychotic episode. Polypharmacy, side effects, many hospitalizations, and suicide were our everyday lives. We knew nothing else-no joy, no holidays. We are working hard to have savings for our son in the future.

We heard about R. when the therapy began, we thought we were in for a beautiful journey of education and refreshment. We got to know TRS better and what mistakes we made in our communication with our son. He found ways to better manage his problems. He was involved in a process of action and improvement. Today he works 2 h a day in the company of our friend.

The parents of a patient composed a letter to RECOVERYTRSGR.

Dear RECOVERYTRSGR,

We lived many years isolated in our house, facing daily problems with our daughter, who suffers from TRS. We were embarrassed; we didn't know what to do. Our family and friendly environment had isolated us. I was ashamed of TRS, for the fact that my child inherited it from her grandfather. It was my fault! I have stigmatized me, my daughter and my family. I preferred to live isolated. It wasn't worth it to seek help.

RECOVERYTRSGR taught me to deal with TRS and accept it as it is. The strategies you taught us helped me reduce the shame and accept TRS as a very serious disability. I eased my guilt, and today I am trying with my daughter to claim her rights.

A patient who participated not in RECOVERYTRSGR and dropped out has also composed a letter to RECOVERYTRSGR:

Dear RECOVERYTRSGR:

I am an orphan, and since I was 18 I have spent most of my time in psychiatric hospitals. A friend of mine introduced you to me. I went and tried to start. I couldn't stand it. Firstly, I didn't have any members of my family next to me. They have died. I found the treatment difficult. I feel very sad and ashamed of TRS. I don't want to meet other people because it will hurt me. I fear treatments and prefer my peace.

A patient who participated in RECOVERYTRSGR but dropped out has chosen to compose a letter to our recovery-oriented therapy:

Dear RECOVERYTRSGR,

My life is exceptionally troublesome with schizophrenia. I was hospitalized many times, and I have changed many psychiatrists. I have heard about RECOVERYTRSGR from another patient.

I visited Dr. Georgila and Dr. Rakitzi, and I decided to participate in this therapy. 190 sessions! I was on edge that I would not be able to do all these 190 sessions! Dr. Georgila clarified to me that we will begin with major changes in my pharmacotherapy, which could help me afterward to do the therapy. Dr. Georgila clarified TRS. After 12 years of schizophrenia, I learned what TRS is! This information made a difference to me in helping me understand how troublesome my mental health disorder is.

My parents have died 5 years ago, and my brother passed away from cancer 1 year ago. The only person who knows about my issue are my uncle, the brother of my mother and his family. This is my family, which supports me. This family participated in psychoeducation at RECOVERYTRSGR. Our communication was moved forward.

I participated in 120 sessions of the program. I felt exceptionally decent, and I attempted to work at the restaurant of my uncle. I was very happy and proud of myself. One day I felt a strong pain in the stomach. I call Dr. Georgila and my internist, and my internist prescribed medical examinations. After 1 week, a cancer diagnosis was made. My parents and my brother died from cancer.

So that was the reason that I didn't continue with RECOVERYTRSGR. It was an enormous dissatisfaction for me. But I have learned to manage with TRS, and this pattern helps me with the cancer diagnosis. I continue with follow-up sessions by Dr. Georgila and Dr. Rakitzi to manage cancer and TRS.

The impressions of our patients with TRS and the three briefs to RECOVERYTRSGR from the patients and the mother display the recovery in process through our program.

It is an honor for us to have met all these people who favored our RECOVERYTRSGR. It is an honor for us to go with them in their troubles, offering a recovery-oriented therapy.

Research studies regarding the effectiveness and efficacy of our therapy are on demand. The combination of clinical implementation and research helps us to realize the genuine needs of our patients and their families and the fitting recovery-oriented programs for these needs.

The following conclusions can be drawn from these briefs or impressions regarding RECOVERYTRSGR:

- It is exceptionally imperative to clarify transparently what TRS is and why it is a particulate category in schizophrenia.
- Pharmacotherapy in TRS is the main therapy and ought to be adjusted appropriately before beginning with evidence-based *psychotherapy.*

- Psychoeducation can help the family understand the challenges of TRS and can offer an alternative way of communication, particularly under negative circumstances.
- The combination of individual and group therapy in RECOVERYTRSGR provides numerous ways to manage resistant cognitive dysfunctions, symptoms, and suicidality. This enhances the plausibility of a sustainable functional outcome and quality of life.
- The cognitive, metacognitive, and recovery perspectives show the leading reply to treatment of TRS and resistant suicidality!
- RECOVERYTRSGR prevents abuse between the family members and teaches people to be assertive toward numerous forms of abuse and malpractice by mental health experts and in life generally.
- RECOVERYTRSGR educates individuals to cope with TRS, and this is a pattern for dealing with other resistant problems in life, such as health and social problems.
- RECOVERYTRSGR displays a democratic therapy, which protects the rights and needs of patients with TRS and their families.
- *RECOVERYTRSGR supports the family of patients with TRS to go from long-term grief, distress, hopelessness, and despair to action for life, hope, and to a better communication.*
- *RECOVERYTRSGR helps patients with TRS and their family to stop the vicious cycle of hospitalizations, suicide, and despair and to find a new way of dealing with TRS that is motivational and recovery-oriented.*
- *RECOVERYTRSGR helps to reduce the stigma because, on the one hand, there is proper psychoeducation for TRS, and on the other hand, it gives the possibility to manage it. Thus the person learns to improve themselves, which improves self-confidence and reduces stigma.*
- *RECOVERYTRSGR is a good answer to the ECT. It is long-term therapy and requires more effort but can improve TRS without side effects.*

Schizophrenia and TRS display chronic mental health disorders. Patients and their families learn to manage with them for their whole lives. A coexistence with a chronic mental health disorder needs long-term professional treatment and evidence-based therapy. The activation of the appropriate resources contributes to a new and positive way of dealing with a severe mental health disorder. RECOVERYTRSGR is able to activate these resources and help people restart their lives in a setting with reasonable objectives.

Mental health experts who choose to work with chronic mental health disorders need good training and education, clinical experience, and the ability to take care of themselves. An education in clinical psychiatry, in clinical psychology, in cognitive behavioral psychotherapy, huge clinical experience with patients with schizophrenia and TRS, and life-long training in programs and psychotherapies for patients with schizophrenia are the suitable conditions to implement RECOVERYTRSGR.

Working with chronic mental health disorders means that experts ought to activate their own resources and find time to do other things, such as entertainment, traveling, spending time with family and friends, and getting to know new cultures. A great psychohygiene activates more motivation in TRS therapy, decreases anxiety, and increases the effectiveness of mental health experts. Schizophrenia and TRS are so universal. So it is exceptionally imperative to get to know also other cultures as well. So it will be awesome when RECOVERYTRSGR is implemented in many nations around the world.

RECOVERYTRSGR presents a marathon achieving improvement and a new restart in life. It is not a marathon to victory, perfectionism, or the total disappearance of problems and inabilities. It is a dynamic program that continues throughout life. It is a dynamic synthesis of ways of dealing with problems and can support not only TRS but also other problems.

RECOVERYTRSGR helps patients with TRS and their families overcome the grief toward a serious mental health disorder. Pharmacotherapy for TRS, psychoeducation, individual and group cognitive behavioral therapy, and rehabilitation present actions which are committed to life and lead to advance and enhancement. This is the best answer to suicidality, chronic disability, weakness, loss of control, and desperation. In other words, the leading reply to anxiety of death as a result of a severe mental health disorder are all the appropriate actions and interventions, which keep patients with TRS alive, living cells of society, and protagonists in their own lives.

If polypharmacy had a voice, what would it say?

The combination of many medications (10 per day) will reduce your stress and give you a chance to sleep better and not fight with positive symptoms. Polypharmacy is quick and can save you from hospitalizations, suicidality, and relapses. You will always be fine!

What would RECOVERYTRSGR answer?

Evidence-based pharmacotherapy highlights clozapine or a better combination of specific agents with clozapine. Ten agents per day bring more problems. Polypharmacy has many side effects and creates problems with my quality of life. Polypharmacy leads me to drop out and increases my hopelessness and the possibility of a new hospitalization.

If non-evidence-based psychotherapies had a voice, what would they say?

We will implement very good therapies; we know they will help you. We feel that.

What would RECOVERYTRSGR answer?

There are evidence-based psychotherapies available, so that can help you.

Many research studies regarding the efficacy of psychotherapy and rehabilitation are available so that you can read them. An evidence-based psychotherapy means that the goal of the interventions is very clear and specific, a manual is available, and efficacy studies as well as meta-analyses are available for us. The effectiveness of a treatment is related to research and not to the feelings of therapists!

If TRS had a voice, what would it say?

I can't sleep, I'm always tense, I eat little, I hear voices, and somebody is watching me and wants to hurt me. People are dangerous, and they have placed microphones in my room and are monitoring me. I want to stay alone without somebody interrupting my routine. I cannot concentrate on anything, and if I cannot solve any problem, I don't want to do anything. I prefer to stay alone at home doing nothing! The only solution for me is suicide-nothing else! (Psychosis)

What would RECOVERYTRSGR answer?

You are tired of non-effective treatments. This led to bad adherence to pharmacotherapy and to relapse. You prefer the psychotic phase because you live with your own "friends"—the hallucinations, the delusions, and the suicidal thoughts. This is your own world. If somebody tries to change your life, you will be aggressive, and you will resist that. But this phase is self-destructive because, you are suicidal and you need hospitalization.

We will make a new restart with the pharmacotherapy, and you will take the x combination, which will improve your sleep, reduce your anxiety, and improve your positive symptoms.

Then we will call your family to psycho-educate them in a new way of communication, which will improve cohesion. They have no right to verbally abuse you, just as you should not be abusive toward your family. Your family will be trained to show more empathy toward you and toward your needs. You will communicate better with each other.

Afterward you will participate in a combination of individual and group cognitive behavioral psychotherapy and rehabilitation that will help you reduce the distress caused by positive and negative symptoms, anxiety, and depression. You will be capable of coping with positive and negative symptoms; your cognitive functions will be improved, as well as your quality of life and functional outcome.

Psychotherapy will help you restructure beliefs related to psychosis, build a program of mood-enhancing activities, and train you in relapse prevention. You will learn to recognize thoughts about yourself.

RECOVERYTRSGR will train you from a recovery perspective. This means that the mental health experts will evaluate your progress with tests, and you will evaluate your progress with your own subjective criteria. This way, there will be an open discussion between the two perspectives, and if there is a disagreement, then you will discuss it openly as it arises.

If grief due to TRS had a voice, what would it say?

I wake up and go to sleep with a big why! Why should I have this disorder? Am I being punished for something? At the beginning, I was shocked as I was hospitalized. I am very angry, and I deny what my doctors and psychotherapists tell me. I feel very tired, I cannot sleep well, and I hear voices all day. Someone is watching me and wants to hurt me. I cannot live with that. I will stop taking my pharmacotherapy, and I will wake up from a bad dream. The truth is me and my life. Everything different from that is not the truth! I will follow my instinct, and my life belongs to me. I don't want to visit psychiatrists and psychotherapists! I don't need any treatment. I will follow what my voices suggest; in other words, live your life without treatment. I would like to have the freedom to do everything I want! Together with my voices!

My grief for my child has deep roots and will never be uprooted! I will live a life of despair and try to find comfort in friends. There is no way out in this life other than deep grief. Anger, denial, depression, hopelessness, and pessimism were my negative emotions. I will not be happy to see my child finish school, study, fall in love, travel, and work. What a shame! What a misfortune!

If RECOVERYTRSGR had a voice, how would it respond to grief?

RECOVERYTRSGR will help you live with more freedom, determination, and autonomy and with a higher quality of life. Your family will have a better psychoeducation regarding TRS; you will be able to control better your voices and delusions that cause distress; you will learn to enhance your mood; you will improve your cognitive functions that lead to a better functional outcome, and finally you will improve your ability to recognize your thoughts about thoughts.

All these strategies show how not to focus on why I have this disorder, but how I can cope with it gaining more control over it! In other words, RECOVERYTRSGR will help you transform the grief regarding TRS into action for life with more hope, autonomy, creativity, determination, and activation for resources! That's real life! So keep going with your therapy with hope and discipline!

RECOVERYTRSGR will help you go through your grief regarding the TRS of your child. You will be an active partner in the therapy. You will support your child through the small changes during treatment. Yes, he/she can travel, he/she can work for a few hours, he/she can fall in love, and she/he can enjoy small, beautiful everyday moments.

If stigma had a voice, what would it say?

The TRS label will mark you forever and leave a mark on you. The stigma you put on yourself and what others put on you. So you will be ashamed and isolated and you will not ask for any help out of shame. You are at a dead end, and society has marginalized you. There is no chance to find a solution. You are a stigma!

If RECOVERYTRSGR had a voice, how would it respond to stigma?

RECOVERYTRSGR gives you the opportunity to get to know TRS better, to learn to manage it with treatments, and to be the protagonist in solving problems. That way, you won't be ashamed of anything. You will be proud of the effort you are making to deal with TRS. Since you know what TRS is and how you are treated, there is no stigma. We all have a right in life to be vulnerable and to be sick!

The best response to stigma is to act for life, communicate with others, and claim from society what belongs to us. Fear, shame, and pessimism have no place in our lives. Be yourself and improve through RECOVERYTRSGR.

If the cognitive perspective had a voice, what would RECOVERYTRSGR say?

I will help you restructure the beliefs associated with vulnerability, weakness, and loss of control (psychosis). This will help you to have control over your hallucinations and delusions, as well as to improve your negative symptoms. Cognitive function will be improved.

If the metacognitive perspective had a voice, what would RECOVERYTRSGR say?

You will be trained to observe thoughts about thoughts and to recognize cognitive distortions. You will have more control over your thoughts, which can reduce your impulsivity, anger, anxiety, and depression.

If the recovery perspective had a voice, what would RECOVERYTRSGR say?

Dr. Rakitzi and Dr. Georgila will evaluate your improvement with psychometric tests (Recovery as an outcome). You, as the protagonist, will evaluate your progress every hour, every day, every week, every month, and every year. You are a valuable partner.

The therapeutic relationship in the context of RECOVERYTRSGR is motivation-, resource-, and recovery-oriented. The advantages and disadvantages of every potential for change and progress will be analyzed. In other words, the therapeutic relationship is a slide to implement changes and improve the quality of life. Thus, patients play a leading role in their own lives through the model of the therapeutic relationship. The therapeutic relationship is an oasis in the desert, where the patients with TRS can rest, relax, and discuss all their problems in a safe environment. Each session of RECOVERYTRSGR gives the opportunity to discuss changes, either for improvements that were made or for unattainable changes. The words change and progress, improvement and achievement of goals are expressed in each session and characterize the therapeutic relationship in RECOVERYTRSGR.

The therapeutic relationship in RECOVERYTRSGR increases motivation for change and progress which simultaneously reduces stigma. The therapeutic relationship is a protection against stigma and isolation because it mobilizes the individual toward change.

The role of the family is very important in RECOVERYTRSGR. The Greek family supports its children in general throughout their lives and much more when they suffer from chronic health problems, such as TRS. Thus, we included in RECOVERYTRSGR a basic cultural element of Greece: the family. Most people with TRS live with their families and enjoy their support. Thus, by including the family in our therapy, we make it a dynamic and decisive element of the treatment, and at the same time, we intervene in it in order to reduce the high expressed emotion toward the patients with TRS.

TRS displays a distinct category of schizophrenia and is one of the most difficult mental health disorders. Patients with TRS should distinguish between themselves and their disorder. They are not the disorder, the TRS. They are people with their own personalities, their own human rights for access to effective treatments, and with the potential to live a life with a better quality of life. They have the right to stand up for themselves and to be assertive toward TRS. But they are not their disorder. They are human beings with the potential for change and improvement!

RECOVERYTRSGR offers the chance to learn to cope with TRS, to be a protagonist in one's life and to fulfill life goals. TRS should not be the biggest obstacle, but a problem like all the others, and with RECOVERYTRSGR goal is possible. Problems should be evaluated as challenges for improvement and progress and as triggers for enhancing the learning potential of patients with TRS and their families. Having a chronic mental health disorder and coping with it proves that the person is very strong and resilient. It is an honor for mental health experts to meet these people and to have cooperated with them.

The value and dignity of human life are guaranteed by the Declaration of Human Rights. Every person has the right to live with dignity, to satisfy his biological and emotional needs, to work, to enjoy his life, and in cases of illness and disability to be able to access effective treatments. Effective treatments must be applied by specialized experts with clinical experience, who will be evaluated in terms of their scientific work. These effective treatments should reach all states of the world, and especially poorer countries.

RECOVERYTRSGR is devoted to the dignity of life and offers alternative ways to dead ends.

The implementation of evidence-based interventions in science to address health problems is also a key criterion for the quality of democracy in any country. The right to health, access to modern treatments, and the protection of our fellow vulnerable citizens are the basic goods of every democracy!

The protection of patients with TRS and their families is a basic obligation of every democratic society. It is not possible to hear that TRS has reached a dead end that the only treatment is ECT, and patients have been abused by non-evidence-based interventions and by mental health experts. If all this is happening, then what quality of democracy do we have?

What is the relationship between democracy and science? Science operates within the framework of democracy and with the rules of democracy. The rights of science stop where its obligations to others, to people, begin. Science has an obligation to produce effective tools and treatments for patients with mental health disorders, and especially with TRS. Science is obliged to be subject to evaluations, and finally it is obliged to ensure all people access to it.

Greece has been going through a socioeconomic crisis from 2008 until today. Greece has many structural problems and does not invest enough funds in the field of health. Our program can fill a gap in the field of mental health in Greece and give the opportunity to patients with TRS and their families to participate at a low cost.

RECOVERYTRSGR will be evaluated in the next few years by us and other colleagues regarding effectiveness and efficacy. We will be exceptionally glad to cooperate with many colleagues from all over the world in order to implement our program. Science is universal and brings people together.

RECOVERYTRSGR was a very beautiful trip for us. The idea for this program began in 2008. This year begins our scientific acquaintance and cooperation in the framework of the implementation of a research protocol on the effectiveness and efficacy of IPT in Greece. The research protocol was implemented in the adult psychiatric department of the G. Gennimatas hospital in Athens. Dr. Georgila was then director of the adult psychiatric department of G. Gennimatas. Enthusiasm for the protocol at the time was great and a structured program for schizophrenia would finally be implemented. During the implementation of the IPT, there was also a sample patient with TRS in which IPT was effective.

The concerns about TRS are just beginning. The IPT was also effective in TRS. But one program was not enough. Thus, through many years of collaboration, the need arose for a comprehensive program just for TRS, in which the family would participate, pharmacotherapy would be best combined with psychotherapy and individual and group therapy would be combined. The combination of various forms of therapy is a better practice of the various functions and enhances socialization.

The sooner TRS is diagnosed, the better. The sooner the appropriate agent is administered, the better. As long as polypharmacy is avoided, the motivation for action for a better quality of life increases. The more interventions we combine, the better!

Our experience has shown that the appropriate pharmacotherapy for TRS needs 2–3 months to act initially. Psychotherapy can afterward begin.

The family plays a crucial role and can destroy or strengthen a positive therapeutic outcome.

Individual cognitive behavioral psychotherapy gives the opportunity to build the therapeutic relationship and reduce suspicion. Skills are slowly practiced, negative beliefs will be restructured, and positive beliefs will be strengthened.

Group therapy provides the opportunity to socialize and learn from others, as well as implement programs to improve cognitive functions, social skills, and problem-solving skills.

The rotation of mental health specialists, the hospitalizations, suicide, and the despair of patients and their families particularly troubled us. The repeating vicious cycle had to be broken.

All the above factors led to the idea of RECOVERYTRSGR. Our program is a result of our clinical experience with TRS and its problems, the above conclusions and the willingness to find an alternative solution to break the vicious cycle of TRS.

The chronic and persistent suicidality of TRS is always difficult for the patients with TRS, their families, and the mental health experts. The thought revolves around the end of life without alternative scenarios and exits and becomes an obsession day and night!

The grief of patients with TRS and their families is an immense cloud over their heads. Psychotic symptoms, depression, and anger dominate throughout the day.

The abusive experiences of our patients with TRS were also painful and difficult for us. These experiences are stored in the memory, which is disturbed when stimuli recall the trauma. Memory dysfunction is expressed through psychotic symptoms.

The comorbidity of TRS with other health problems, such as cancer, proves that patients with TRS need help to deal with TRS, so that they can be able also to deal with other health problems.

TRS is associated with stigma. Patients and their families have been ashamed for many years and live in isolation. They do not dare to speak and claim their rights. They live immersed in their stigma and what society puts on them.

Stigma is a very big and fundamental problem in mental health disorders and especially in TRS. The person with TRS is heavily stigmatized through the vicious cycle of the disorders, ashamed of the problems, isolated, has many relapses and has no motivation to seek help.

Our patients and their families, our clinical experience, and all the above findings brought us to the idea of creating a structured treatment for TRS. Our discussions about these issues in the context of peer supervision and our concern about

TRS led us to RECOVERYTRSGR. 2021 was the year of the first discussions, and today with this book, our vision is slowly becoming a reality, and we are very grateful to Springer Nature.

The 190 sessions lay the foundation for a proper initiation in the context of pharmacotherapy, for the application of a wide range of psychotherapies, for a combination of psychotherapies, and for cooperation with the family. This is how individual and group interventions are combined with all their advantages, and the vicious cycle of TRS can be broken.

Breaking the vicious circle of TRS leads to a bright light in the tunnel, with the prospect of getting out of it to see beautiful landscapes and an endless blue sea. There is a prospect in this life for something better, there is a prospect to better manage the positive and negative symptoms, anxiety and depression, and finally, cognitive functions can be improved. All of these have a positive impact on functional outcome and quality of life.

RECOVERYTRSGR can also lead to a reduction in stigma because people learn to manage their problem more comfortably by setting limits to any form of stigma. In other words, the best way to deal with stigma is to develop mental health resilience in the face of the problem, which RECOVERYTRSGR achieves.

The pilot application of RECOVERYTRSGR showed us the way to further research its effectiveness and efficacy of it. Patients with TRS built a more durable therapeutic relationship with us and improved symptoms, cognitive functions, functioning, and recovery.

They felt that for the first time in their lives, they dared to manage this traumatic situation, TRS. They can be in control and try daily to improve any malfunctions. They are the protagonists in their lives and in our lives.

Patients with TRS and families go through grief, despair, and suicidality in a constant effort to recover and reintegrate into society. They define their lives and set new goals. They are in recovery during their whole life! This makes their lives different, vivid, and challenging, which is an important protective mechanism against suicidality.

The ability to repeat this treatment due to relapse is also a very important feature and advantage. They are given time and space to fall back into a secure frame.

Patients with TRS and their families need time to learn new things through RECOVERYTRSGR and try to slowly integrate them into their daily lives. The scope of our treatment is slowly generalizing to other goals, such as managing organic health problems or some kind of loss.

Mental health experts feel that through this structured program, that they have the time and space to implement their therapy by building a better therapeutic relationship with patients with TRS and their families. They have time to monitor them systematically and under all conditions. In this way, a better empathy for the sufferers will be developed.

The development of an integrative recovery-oriented program is due to many factors and above all a common vision for more democracy in mental health, and of solving problems of chronic mental disorders with more flexibility, team spirit, and long-term interventions.

The therapy of patients with TRS displays a very rich clinical and human experience. Without them, we would not have proceeded with the creation of this program. It is our honor to have met them, to have worked with them, and to have spent endless therapeutic hours with difficult but also pleasant moments!

The continuation of the application of RECOVERYTRSGR to other patients with TRS and their families, as well as the training of other colleagues in our program, is our first priority the next few years!

Science has given us the opportunity to find new dimensions in modern therapies, and we should be grateful for that. We are even more grateful to our patients because developing a therapy would not be possible without the presence and contributions of people with TRS and their families.

Ultimately, transforming weak, suspicious, suicidal, and socially isolated individuals with TRS into active people, open to new life experiences, with new meaning to their lives and integrating into society by claiming all their rights, is one of the greatest experience for all mental health professionals.

Eleni's letter to TRS will be presented:

Dear TRS,

I have learned to live with you since I was 17 years old. I have been hospitalized ten times to date. The vicious cycle of schizophrenia and TRS was a nightmare for me. Suicidality, discontinuation of pharmacotherapy, change of mental health experts, and aggression in the family are my daily routine. I'm creating problems for my family!

My parents heard about a new treatment in Athens. At first, I didn't think I could be helped. The TRS monster won't leave me alone. I also did ECT. It didn't help! I got worse. I don't want anything anymore, I'm tired. I promised that I would make one last attempt regarding TRS. I was and am very ashamed of my problems.

Eleni has participated on RECOVERYTRSGR and expressed the following impressions:

When I heard that I had to do 190 sessions, I was scared. It is very tiring. When I heard that my family would be included, I was scared too. We dont have good interfamiliar relations at all. But how do I get out of the vicious circle of TRS. So let's try.

Dr. Georgila explained TRS to me and suggested a change in agents. I was taking seven agents a day. It took about 3 months to balance. Then the collaboration with the family began. We expressed what bothers us and the aggression stopped. Afterward the psychotherapies began! I felt like I was improving some things step by step and I could be in control. I am still in the recovery process. RECOVERYTRSGR is for me, a family where everything is discussed!

So Eleni describes very well her dead end in the last 10 years. The vicious cycle of TRS: Polypharmacy and hospitalizations. Helen was now suspicious of the mental health system. She decided to participate on RECOVERYTRSGR.

Dr. Georgila's letter to TRS,

Dear TRS,

Schizophrenia and TRS were and is for me a daily routine of my work. I can't do without it. The TRS is greater in percentages than we imagined.

Your vicious cycle of suicidality, relapses, discontinuation of agents, and constant changes of mental health experts has tired and saddened me many times.

Worst of all was polypharmacy, with many side effects for patients with TRS. But I learned to deal with you. I have been giving clozapine from the beginning, which is very effective for TRS. I also trained many mental health experts in it. So there is a way to deal with TRS. But we need new agents for TRS. I also propose long-term psychotherapy.

I was shocked many years ago by the story of a woman with TRS, who was also sexually abused. The dual trauma of TRS and abuse was in front of me in every session. I couldn't avoid it. I helped this lady quite effectively, and I also suggested cognitive behavioral psychotherapy.

The stigma of TRS is a very big problem. People remained untreated and isolated for many years because of their shame. Thus precious time was lost.

I am optimistic about the future of pharmacotherapy regarding TRS. There are also very effective psychotherapies available.

Dr. Georgila's letter to RECOVERYTRSGR,

Dear RECOVERYTRSGR,

The idea of developing a therapy for TRS gave me great joy and optimism. RECOVERYTRSGR makes it possible step by step to build a therapeutic relationship of trust and security. Pharmacotherapy is discussed from the first moment, and all the difficulties of the past are analyzed. We are making a new beginning with the agents.

The family will be included. This is very important because family plays a crucial role in the life of patients with TRS. Individual and group cognitive behavioral psychotherapy are being implemented in a long term. This gives us the opportunity to arm our patients with skills to reintegrate into society more quickly. Thus, stigma is reduced, and functionality and self-confidence are improved.

Thank you for giving me the opportunity to help my patients in a structured and long-term way.

Dr. Rakitzi's letter to TRS,

Dear TRS,

I was confronted with TRS years ago. At that time, I didn't have enough clinical experience. I was scared and referred the patient to the hospital. I am saddened by the stigma you leave on patients with TRS and their families, their grief and your complexity. The stigma among these patients is very large and deep. They stay for many years without treatment because they are ashamed.

Today I feel safer with TRS. I know the difficulties, how I have to increase their motivation, and that suicide is the first priority in the treatment. I also know that clozapine is a very effective agent.

Your vicious cycle makes me angry, saddens me, and, at the same time, motivates me to break it psychotherapeutically. The priority is the right pharmacotherapy, and after the patient is stabilized, psychotherapies can be applied. There are ways to deal with it.

Dr. Rakitzi's letter to RECOVERYTRSGR,

Dear RECOVERYTRSGR,

I am very happy to participate in the development of this recovery-oriented treatment program. It is a systematic program that combines pharmacotherapy, individual and group psychotherapy. This variety of interventions can manage the complex problems of TRS at all levels.

Improvement in symptoms, cognitive functions, and thinking leads to improvements in functional outcome and quality of life. Chronic grief turns into action for life, and the stigma is replaced by the confidence to accept and defend myself as I am!

I am optimistic with you that we will powerfully help many patients with TRS. We will make it. If anything counts in this life, it is action for life.

This action also makes sense to me because I can effectively help my vulnerable fellow citizens with more than 80% disability.

What I love about therapy is its ability to holistically intervene with suicidality, grief, and stigma. Acting for life washes away all that misery and isolation. The stigma in particular is deeply rooted in TRS since it appears from the first moment problems manifest and from the first acute psychotic episode. It's like a trauma!

RECOVERYTRSGR gives us the possibility to break the vicious cycle of TRS by reducing the stigma and grief and strengthening the relationships with the family and the personal development of the patient with TRS. Thank you for this beautiful trip.

I will continue this effort with you at every opportunity. This is how we will reduce the suicidality of these people to a minimum, and we will integrate them into society.

All the best for all of us!

Over 30% of patients with schizophrenia belong to TRS. This led to the need to create a specialized program for TRS. This category is the most difficult and needs specific therapeutic strategies. It is the category that creates frustration and hopelessness.

The TRS carries a very heavy load. They have a very deep stigma and isolate themselves from society. They are overwhelmed and do not ask for help from the experts. Interfamily relationships are often disturbed. Their grief, which manifests itself in psychotic symptoms, is also very deep and lasting. They often face traumas, such as physical, sexual, and psychological abuse. These traumas reinforce grief as well as stigma.

The above load presupposes the structured and evidence-based treatment of TRS. The therapeutic relationship combined with interventions can be a springboard to deal with the disorder and then the rest, such as trauma, grief, and stigma. RECOVERYTRSGR is a long-term action for life that gives the right to leave with dignity, proud, and assertiveness.

RECOVERYTRSGR gives TRS a chance. It reduces frustration, increases hope, and intervenes on all levels. It respects the patients with TRS and their family. RECOVERYTRSGR protects against abuse and constitutes a democratic framework for intervention. Its duration is long term, and this can be tiring, but on the other hand, TRS is only treated long-term and with a combination of interventions.

RECOVERYTRSGR gives a basic message of life in TRS, but also in any chronic mental health disorder. There are problems and obstacles with malfunctions in everyday life. There is the grief, the stigma, and the trauma. But there is also a structured response for action to life. RECOVERYTRSGR gives inspiration to patients with TRS because it focuses on their problems by accepting them and changing life conditions.

RECOVERYTRSGR confronts action for life against misery, powerlessness, and vulnerability. It inspires mental health experts, and patients with TRS and their families to work cohesive, optimistic, motivation-, recovery-, and resource-oriented against mystery, vulnerability, and weakness.

We wish you a nice trip RECOVERYTRSGR and we hope to inspire many of our colleagues all over the world! Time will show if RECOVERYTRSGR completes its journey and fulfills the basic goals of a recovery-oriented therapy. We are very happy to make available to the scientific community a new, modern, and recovery-oriented therapy for the patients with TRS and their families.

Competing Interests The authors have no conflicts of interest to declare that are relevant to the content of this chapter.

Ethical Approval Our case studies follow the ethical standards of the 1964 Declaration of Helsinki and its amendments. Informed consent to publish was obtained from individual participants.

GPSR Compliance

The European Union's (EU) General Product Safety Regulation (GPSR) is a set of rules that requires consumer products to be safe and our obligations to ensure this.

If you have any concerns about our products, you can contact us on ProductSafety@springernature.com

In case Publisher is established outside the EU, the EU authorized representative is:

Springer Nature Customer Service Center GmbH
Europaplatz 3
69115 Heidelberg, Germany

Batch number: 10732119

Printed by Printforce, the Netherlands